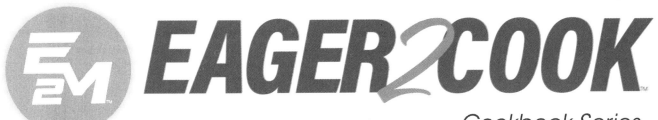

EAGER2COOK

Cookbook Series

Healthy Recipes for Healthy Living

Beef & Poultry

SPARK Publications
Charlotte, North Carolina

Eager 2 Cook™: Healthy Recipes for Healthy Living
Beef & Poultry
E2M Chef Connect LLC

Eager 2 Cook™ series by Golden Spoon Holdings, LLC

The E2M program provides suggestions on eating a whole food diet that has successfully helped tens of thousands of members achieve their weight loss goals. Before you start this or any program, consult with your physician to clear if this program is a fit for you, your body, and your health, taking into account allergies, pregnancy, or any other physical condition. The content in this book is intended to be generally informative and not provide medical or nutritional advice, and has not been evaluated by physicians, nutritionists, or the Food and Drug Administration (FDA). The E2M program makes no healing claims and does not guarantee any health or weight loss successes. Resulting meals depend on preparation and ingredients used, and the E2M program or cookbooks make no warranty regarding the outcome of your use of these recipes.

Designed, produced, and published by
SPARK Publications
SPARKpublications.com
Charlotte, North Carolina

Written by: Chef Jennie Casselman and Chef Andres Chaparro

Photography by: Shane Amoroson

Printed in the United States of America

Paperback, December 2022, ISBN: 978-1-953555-40-3
eBook, December 2022, ISBN: 978-1-953555-41-0

Library of Congress Control Number: 9781953555403

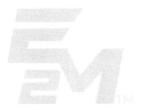

Dedication

I dedicate this book to all the people who believed in me. With positive support anything is possible, and the people in my life who support my wild ideas give me the fuel to chase my dreams each day. I would not be successful without you. Thank you.

Jeff Witherspoon

Table of
Contents

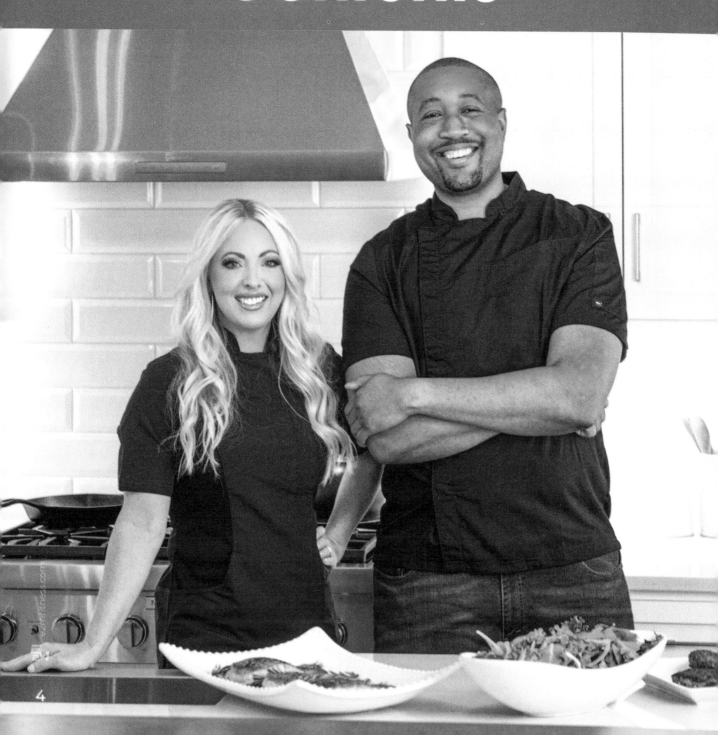

4

Beef

Turkey

Chicken

Dressings

Spice Blends

Journals & Checklists

Introduction to
E2M™ Fitness

What is the E2M™ Program?

It is a virtual, eight-week, rapid body transformation program for adults, which consists of workouts, meal plans, cooking classes, mental fitness, and personal coaching. Workouts are designed for all levels and abilities and can be done at home or a gym. Meal plans vary from week to week and are free of supplements, using only whole, nutrient-dense foods. Our meal plans can accommodate any dietary restrictions, including postpartum recovery and vegan. Each member gains access to certified fitness coaches and thousands of other program members who make up our fitness community. Our Fit Family is made up of people across the world from various backgrounds and age demographics, but what we have in common is one goal: to encourage each other to reach our personal best lifestyle and fitness goals. And after the first eight weeks, the program is available for free to maintain progress.

This isn't about getting "skinny" or "beach ready"; it's about building a healthier lifestyle, living longer, and getting the most out of the body you've been given. This is a lifestyle of health and wellness, and we have the tools to support you in every step of your journey. Whether you want to lose a few pounds, tone up and get stronger, or learn how to sustain a healthier lifestyle with your family, we'd love to help you.

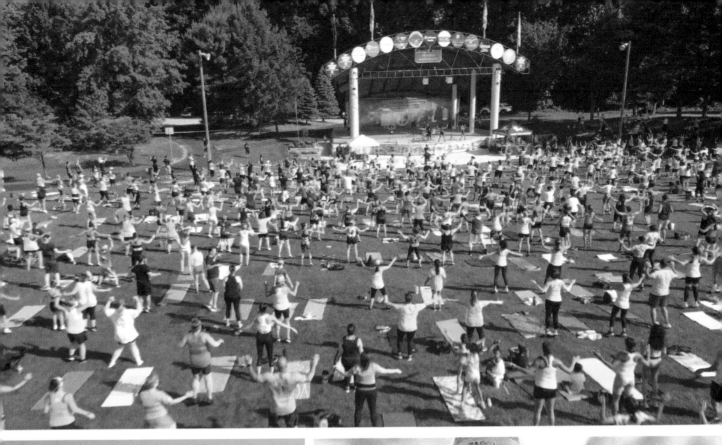

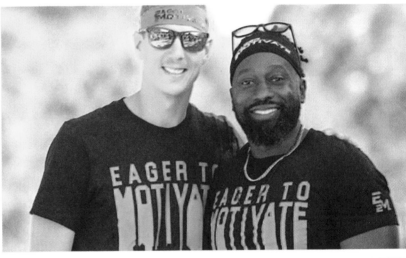

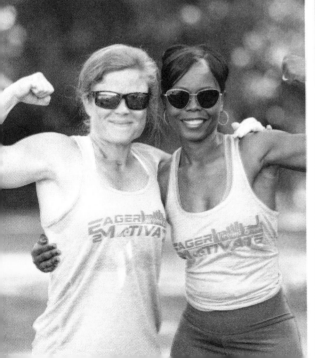

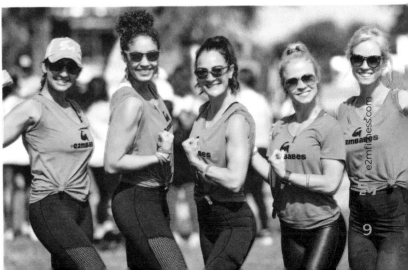

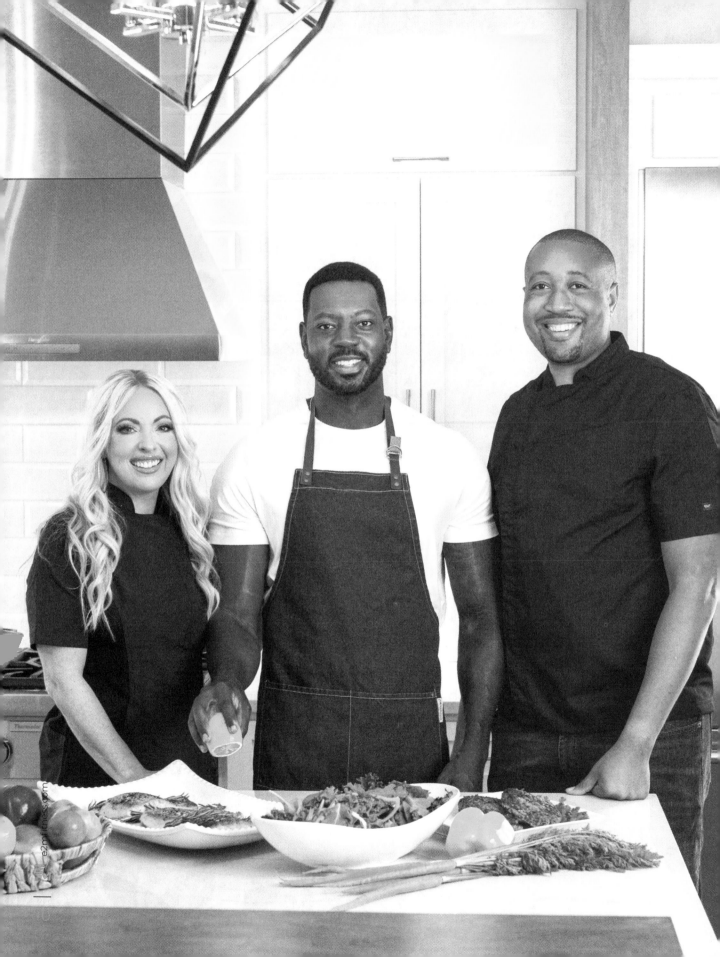

Note to
Members

To my amazing E2M fitness family, we did it!

This cookbook would not be possible without you. It is my sincere hope that this cookbook becomes another tool you can use to maintain your health for years to come. The chefs put lots of time into this and I am excited to see even better results now that you can be a little more creative and still stay on plan. Cooking can be time consuming, but learning to love the process of preparing healthy meals to fuel your body can make cooking your new hobby.

These cookbooks are for us but not only for us, so feel free to recommend the cookbooks to your family and friends because they need to eat healthy too, and they just might end up joining the E2M family. As you improve your health, your life will also improve. JUST KEEP TRYING. Finally, thank you to our amazing chefs Jennie and Andres! They wanted to share some E2M community favorite recipes, and some new ones, in a usable format to make life easier and being healthy more enjoyable. I hope you love what we put together.

Jeff Witherspoon

"It is my goal to help as many people as possible, and I can't wait to help you improve your health, improve your life! I look forward to the chance to be your guide on your journey to your optimal health and fitness."

– JEFF WITHERSPOON

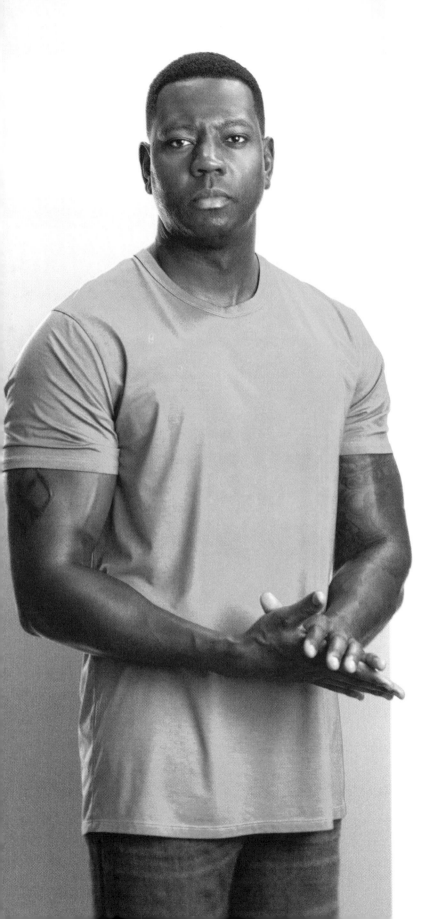

Jeff Witherspoon

Owner, Founder

Jeff Witherspoon's fitness journey began when he was a young athlete at The Citadel in Charleston, South Carolina. Jeff received a full-ride scholarship and worked without ceasing to quickly become a champion track-and-field athlete. He found great joy in bringing home numerous wins for the Bulldogs.

Upon graduation, Jeff began a successful career in the army as a field artillery officer; he has served our country in several overseas tours. While on a deployment, he found fitness as a way to cope with the stresses of combat. He enjoyed not only the way that working out made his body look but also the way that focusing on his health made him feel. Jeff found that "fitness became a place of release and therapy." Fitness enabled him to manage high levels of stress in the military and to handle more stress in a positive way.

Later in his career, Jeff became a certified hand-to-hand combat instructor for the army. This certification and practice introduced him to another form of fitness and discipline that he also enjoyed. This new level of discipline would eventually permeate all areas of his life.

As Jeff began to encourage fellow soldiers and friends to work out and eat healthy, he recognized his passion to help others. Fitness and nutrition became tools he used to help lead other soldiers with PTSD in coping with day-to-day stressors and to assist them in improving their overall health and wellness. This sparked his desire to become a certified personal trainer.

Jeff's passion and business grew as he began to see how his knowledge and motivation were helping others transform their lives. Providing accurate and factual advice to improve others' fitness levels is his main goal. Through all his experiences, he strategically created what is now E2M Fitness, a worldwide fitness program changing lives one day at a time.

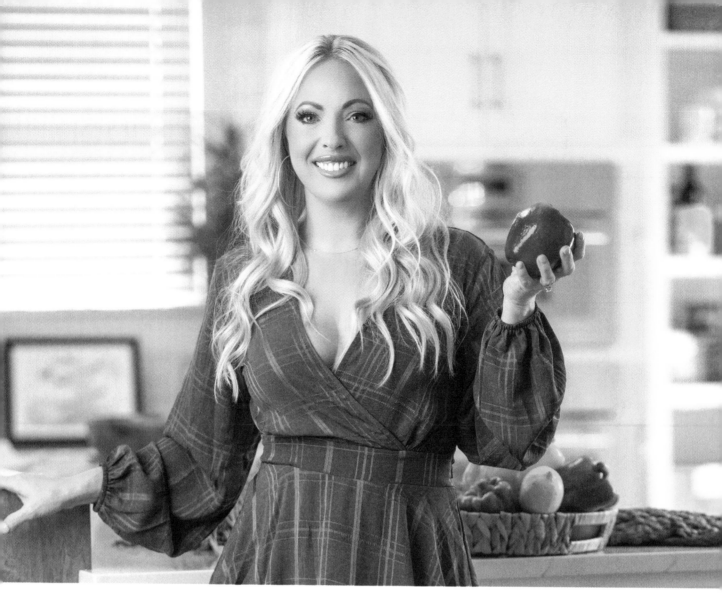

Jennie Casselman

Chef & NASM Certified Nutrition Coach

Growing up in a large southern family, Jennie always enjoyed being in the kitchen with her mom. "I was raised in a family who honored dinnertime. My mom would cook from scratch every night, and then we would all sit around the dinner table and talk about our day." Jennie appreciated all the hard work and commitment it took from her parents to be able to maintain this special tradition for their family.

Her passion for nutrition and food didn't become clear until her late twenties when she was diagnosed with melanoma. "It was a very scary time in my life, but I knew that I could make better decisions for my overall health." She started learning about nutrition and holistic health, which led her to culinary school.

Jennie started her career in nutrition and food service after graduating from Johnson & Wales University in Charlotte, North Carolina. She spent over ten years working in the corporate food service management industry. She trained chefs across the country on how to write nutritious menus for clients of all ages from birth to retirement.

With a background in cheer and dance, Jennie has always enjoyed staying active. She continues to stay active now with E2M workouts and enjoys hiking with her husband and twins. Jennie joined the E2M staff as one of the chefs in November 2020 and has enjoyed teaching online cooking classes and being a part of every life that has been transformed by this program. "My heart's desire is to continue to educate others and share how to fuel your body, as well as to emphasize that healthy can be delicious!"

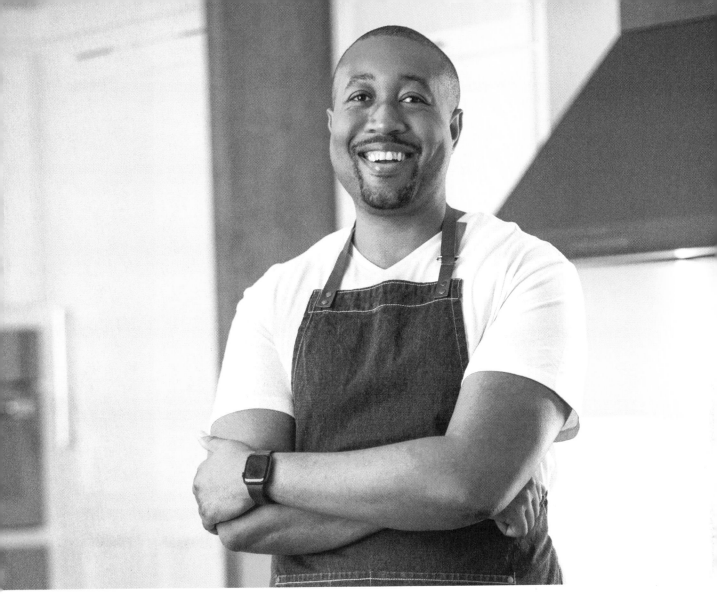

Andres Chaparro

Chef

Since he was young, Andres has always been involved with cooking. He started his career as an intern for a small bakery in his hometown. This gave him a little taste of the industry, which was all he needed to realize that he wanted to pursue a culinary career. After receiving formal training from Johnson & Wales University in Charlotte, North Carolina, he began working and gaining experience in kitchens from coast to coast. With over thirteen years of experience in the food service industry, he looks forward to bringing healthy cooking back to the main screen.

Andres first joined the E2M program in 2018 as a community member, which started his love of running. At the end of 2020, Andres transitioned to the E2M staff by providing weekly online cooking classes. Andres has enjoyed teaching countless E2M members how to make simple, healthy, and flavorful food.

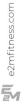

"Trust the Process™"

– JEFF WITHERSPOON

E2M™ Fitness
Success Stories

The jaw-dropping before and after photos of our clients are a direct result of following the E2M Fitness meal and exercise program.

The meal plan includes the recipes in all of our cookbooks written by the chefs of E2M Fitness.

Learning how to fuel your body with nutrient-dense proteins, vegetables, and healthy fats is the key to transitioning to a healthier lifestyle. With proper nutrition and exercise you can change your lifestyle! Healthy recipes and healthy habits lead to healthy living.

Success stories are shared throughout this cookbook. To learn more about the fitness program, please visit E2Mfitness.com

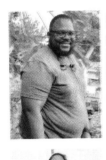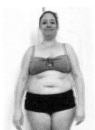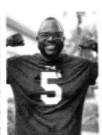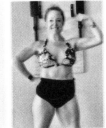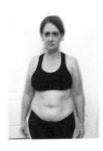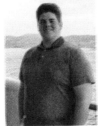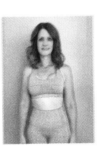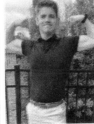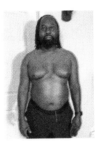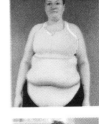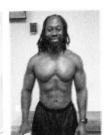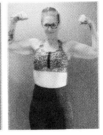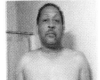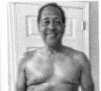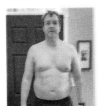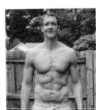

Meal Prep
Strategy

Why is meal prep so important?

Meal prep has become increasingly popular not only for those with busy schedules but also for those looking to eat healthier. Having healthy options readily available helps to manage cravings and to prevent you from making impulsive choices. Follow some of these time-saving strategies to help ditch the last-minute drive-thru and the extra expense of takeout.

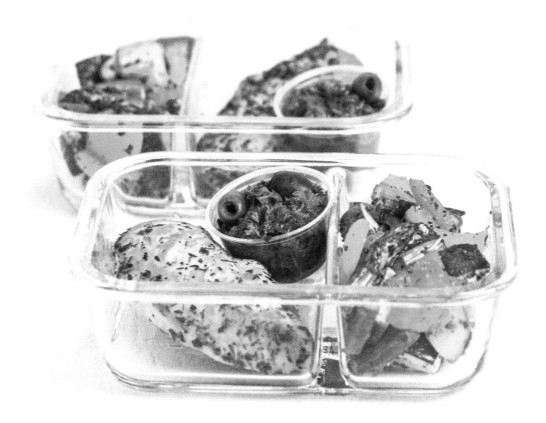

Meal Prep

Meal prep simply means preparing ingredients or whole meals in advance to save you time and set yourself up for success. It can be as simple as washing and chopping vegetables to be ready to cook on those busy weeknights. It can also be cooking and assembling entire meals that can be quickly heated and served for you or your whole family. Chopping vegetables or preparing meal components like your protein will save you time and energy, which we can all use more of during our busy seasons of life. Planned leftovers are another simple strategy to make sure you have healthy choices on hand. When you are preparing one recipe, simply make an extra serving to ensure you have another meal ready to take with you to work the next day. Spending a little extra time in the kitchen once or twice a week preparing your meal components is the key to a successful meal plan strategy.

Meal Prep Containers

Be sure to have plenty of storage containers with airtight lids to maintain quality and freshness. You can use glass or BPA-free plastic containers. For larger batch cooking and freezer meals, foil pans work great. Gallon-size ziplock bags and mason jars are ideal for storage. A vacuum sealer is a great option for preserving large amounts of prepared food, allowing food to remain safe for up to several months in the freezer.

Meal Prep Planning

Choose the recipes you would like to prepare for three to four days of meals. Try to select recipes that use similar ingredients to help reduce your grocery bill. Also check your local grocery store ads and farmers market to buy items that are on sale and seasonally available. You can use the **E2M Weekly Meal Planner** (see checklist pages) to track your recipes and make your grocery list based on your weekly meal plan. Then go to the store!

Grocery Shopping Tips:

1. Print and bring your weekly meal list.

2. Decide on which proteins you would like to prepare.

3. Choose two to three recipes you would like to make and select vegetables and fats to compliment the protein.

4. When shopping, stick to the perimeter of the store. Most of your fresh produce, proteins, and healthy fats are located on the outer perimeter of a grocery store. The inner aisles typically contain prepackaged foods that are not the most nutritious options available. Frozen and canned vegetables are also great options and another great way to meal prep.

5. Dry spices and herbs add loads of flavor to produce and proteins, so be sure to stock your spice cabinet with a variety of spices, including sea salt and black pepper!

6. Double check food labels and ingredients to make sure there are no added sugars or ingredients that you cannot pronounce!

7. Only buy enough for three to four days so you do not waste food that may spoil quickly, such as fresh meats and produce.

   Now you are ready to get in the kitchen and start cooking! Always be sure to read the entire recipe to ensure you are following the steps in order and you have all your ingredients. Enjoy prepping!

Food
Safety

As you embark on your journey and getting back into the kitchen, it is important to know some basic food safety guidelines not only for yourself but also those you will be serving. Food safety plays a big part in your overall health journey. Germs can live in many conditions, so it is important to wash your produce, hands, utensils, and surfaces often while preparing food.

Wash Hands and Surfaces Often

- Never prep raw meat and vegetables on the same cutting board.
- Do not rinse or wash raw meat, seafood, or eggs.
- Did you know that the easiest way to prevent the spread of germs is to properly wash your hands? This is important and needs to be done any time that you are preparing different items in your kitchen. For example, you would need to wash your hands after you touch any uncooked proteins, ready-to-eat items, and vegetables.
- Properly washing your cutting boards with hot, soapy water after preparing each food item and before you go on to the next item is critical. This reduces the spread of germs and the risk of cross contamination.
- Chef Andres and Chef Jennie prefer to use separate cutting boards for proteins and vegetables. Plastic cutting boards are great for meat and wooden is best for vegetables and fruits. Wood boards are porous and can increase the likelihood of cross contamination.

Refrigerate and Store Properly

- As you start this journey into a healthier you, it may be tempting to overshop and pack your refrigerator with healthy items. It is important to not overstock your refrigerator. You need to allow adequate airflow to move throughout and keep the temperature around 40 degrees.
- Refrigerate perishable items like proteins within 2 hours of shopping.
- The freezer will be more efficient if kept full and if the top shelf is not crowded. Just like in the fridge, adequate airflow is critical.
- To prevent cross-contamination, do not store pre-cooked or plant-based "meat" next to raw meat. Wash and rinse all fresh produce before storing it in the fridge.
- Store raw meats and poultry at the bottom of the refrigerator to prevent cross-contamination with produce.

Temperature Control and Reheating

- Did you know there is a safe way to store your prepared meals and reheat them? The most important step of proper storage is not letting the meals stay out at room temperature for a long time before placing them in the refrigerator. When storing the meals in the refrigerator, place the food into smaller 1"-2" deep, airtight containers and ensure the lid is not tightly secured. This will allow steam from the food to
- escape and adequately cool before placing the lid on and completing this process.
- When reheating your prepared meals, the Centers for Disease Control and Prevention recommends allowing food to reach to 165 degrees. When using a microwave, stir food halfway through cooking.
- By taking these steps, you are heading in the right direction regarding your food safety.

Cooking
Basics

Roasting and Baking
(325 to 450 degrees)

Roasting and baking are similar types of dry-heat cooking methods that use hot air to cook food. Roasting and baking at 325 to 450 degrees will brown the surface of the food, which will enhance the flavor. Roasting is a cooking method that can be done on sheet pans or roasting dishes. Chef Jennie prefers to roast on sheet pans covered with parchment paper to make for easy cleanup.

Roasting and baking are done in a standard oven. This technique cooks food evenly, at the same heat and at the same time. Roasting and baking require food be cooked uncovered to allow hot, dry air to circulate freely around the food. Proteins and vegetables can easily be cooked together with this technique. Be sure not to overcrowd your pan by putting food too close together. You want the air to circulate around the food to give it a nice crispy outside.

A meat thermometer is an extremely helpful tool to figure out the internal temperature of your protein and to know when it is a safe temperature for consuming. Cooking times can vary depending on equipment, so the use of a meat thermometer is the most exact way to find the internal temperature.

Cooking Tip: Prepare food for roasting and baking by cutting it into similar sizes so it cooks evenly.
Cooking Tip: Cover your sheet pan with parchment paper to clean up easily and to preserve the surface of the pans longer.

Broiling
(500 degrees)

Broiling is also a dry-heat cooking method that requires the food to be close to the heat source. This will cook the surface of the food quickly as well as brown the surface for more flavor. Chef Jennie and Chef Andres like to finish off dishes, especially chicken and fish, with two to three minutes under the broiler to enhance the flavors already used for the foods.

Cooking Tip: Stay close by when broiling; it only takes the broiler a few minutes before it can burn your food.

Grilling
(high heat)

Grilling simply means heating the food from below with high heat, whether using a gas, charcoal, or indoor grill. The food is typically only turned one time during the cooking process, giving the food the ever-so-desired grill marks. Grilling can also be achieved with a grill pan or grill grate that goes over a gas stove top. As with most cooking methods, it is important to heat the grill before adding the food and to make sure your grill grates are clean. Rather than oiling the pans or grates as you would with other cooking methods, oil your food directly when grilling.

Fish, chicken, vegetables, and fruit are better off being cooked at a lower temperature on the grill for a longer time.

Safety Tip: Always make sure the tools you use with a grill are specific for grilling and can stand up to high heat.

Sauté
(low to medium heat)

Sautéing is one of the most common ways to cook protein and vegetables at home. It is a quick cooking method that requires a little oil and a wide shallow pan. A helpful tip for sautéing food evenly is to not overcrowd your pan with too much food. Overcrowding can cause the heat to decrease and create steam that would end up steaming your food instead of sautéing it. To sauté food and make sure it cooks evenly, you can toss the food in the pan, then flip or move it around with a spatula. Think *Top Chef* or hibachi chef tricks!

It is important to allow your pan to heat up before adding a small amount of oil that has a high smoke point. Extra-virgin olive oil has a lower smoke point and will burn quickly. Allow the cooking oil to heat for a minute before adding the ingredients to the pan. Chef Jennie's and Chef Andres's recommended cooking oils are avocado oil and coconut oil spray.

Safety Tip: If using spray oils, please do not use over an open flame. Spray the pan prior to turning on a gas stove top.

Steaming and Boiling

Steaming and boiling are both low-fat cooking methods that do not require cooking oil. They do cook food at higher temperatures since the water needs to be boiling, but the indirect heat is what cooks the food during steaming. You will need a deep-sided pot and a steaming basket. Make sure to put enough water in the pot so that it doesn't evaporate out, but not too much to cause it to boil over. Most vegetables are excellent options for food for steaming and boiling.

Cast-Iron Skillet

Stove Top Cooking with Cast-Iron: Cast-iron's ability to absorb and distribute heat evenly makes it one of the best cooking vessels. Allow the cast-iron skillet to come to temperature by putting it over the heat for five to ten minutes to thoroughly heat. Once it reaches the desired temperature, it can consistently hold that temperature for an extended period of time, allowing you to cook your food evenly.

Chef Andres says, "When it comes to different cuts of meat, the best cooking process is a combination of both high- and low-temperature cooking methods." A cast-iron skillet is the perfect vessel for this method. Elevated temperatures sear and caramelize the outside, giving it the perfect outer crust to your protein. Chef Jennie loves to sear chicken and beef at a high heat to start and then finish off the cooking in the oven. Chef Jennie prefers to use her cast-iron skillet for most cooking methods!

Grilling with Cast-Iron: Fish and vegetables can be challenging to grill since they are delicate. Using a cast-iron pan or griddle allows you to get that over-the-fire flavor without losing your food between the grates.

Safety and Care of Cast-Iron: Cast-iron skillets require particular care but are worth it and will last for decades! Cleaning cast-iron is easy. Avoid harsh detergents and soaps. If food is cooked onto the surface, add water and turn on the heat to bring it to a simmer. Use a wooden spoon to scrape the food from the pan and rinse. Once the skillet is clean and completely dry, rub it with a small amount of high-temperature oil—like avocado oil or coconut oil—to prevent rusting. This last step is the most important, according to Chef Jennie: don't forget to "season" your cast-iron skillet to prevent rust.

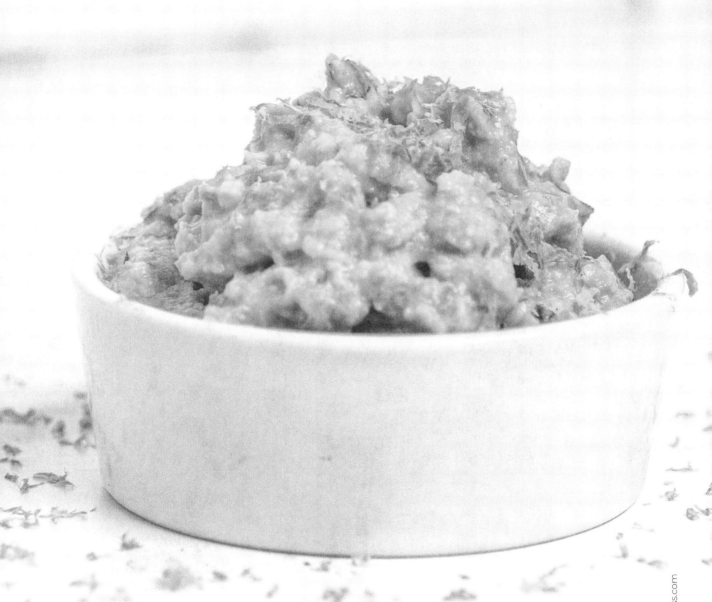

Meet the
Certified Trainers

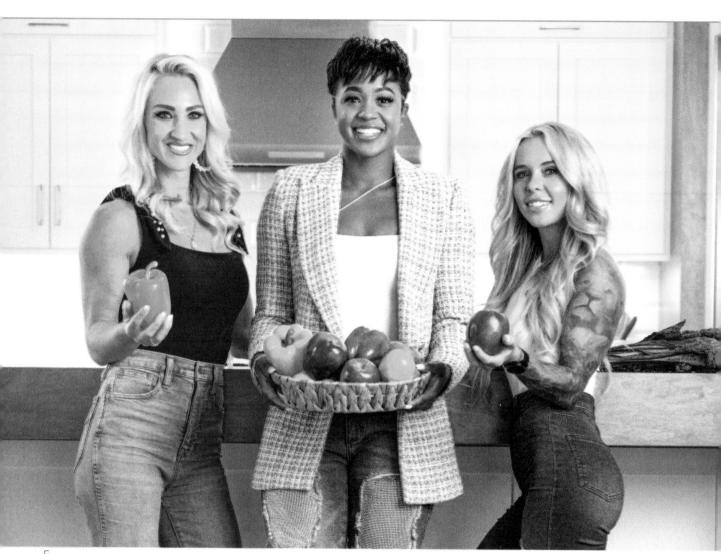

Mandy

"Fitness is
all-or-something,
not all-or-nothing"

Alicia

"Your GOAL is your destination!
Your ACTIONS are your vehicle!
CONSISTENCY and DISCIPLINE
are your fuel! Enjoy the journey
as much as the destination"

Whit

"The body
achieves what
the mind believes"

Suggested
Kitchen Tools

Measuring Tools

Digital scale

Measuring cups

Measuring spoons

Meat thermometer

Utensils

Tongs

Rubber and metal spatulas

Wooden spoon

Zester/Microplane

Sharp knife

Vegetable peeler

Can opener

Citrus juicer

Plastic cutting board
(best for proteins)

Wood cutting board
(best for fruits and vegetables)

Cooking Vessels

Cast-iron skillet

Sauté pan

Sheet pans

Roasting pans

Grill (gas or charcoal)

Grill pan for indoor grilling

Air fryer

Steaming basket

Other
Suggested Items

Heat-resistant gloves or towels

Oven mitts

Salad spinner

Colander

E2M apron

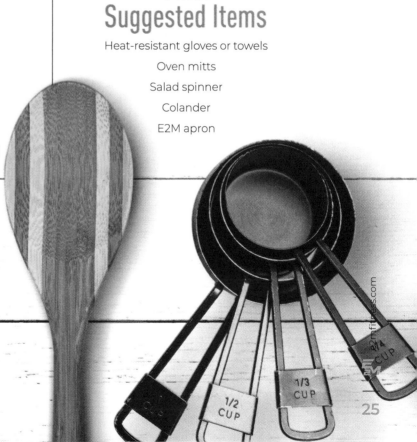

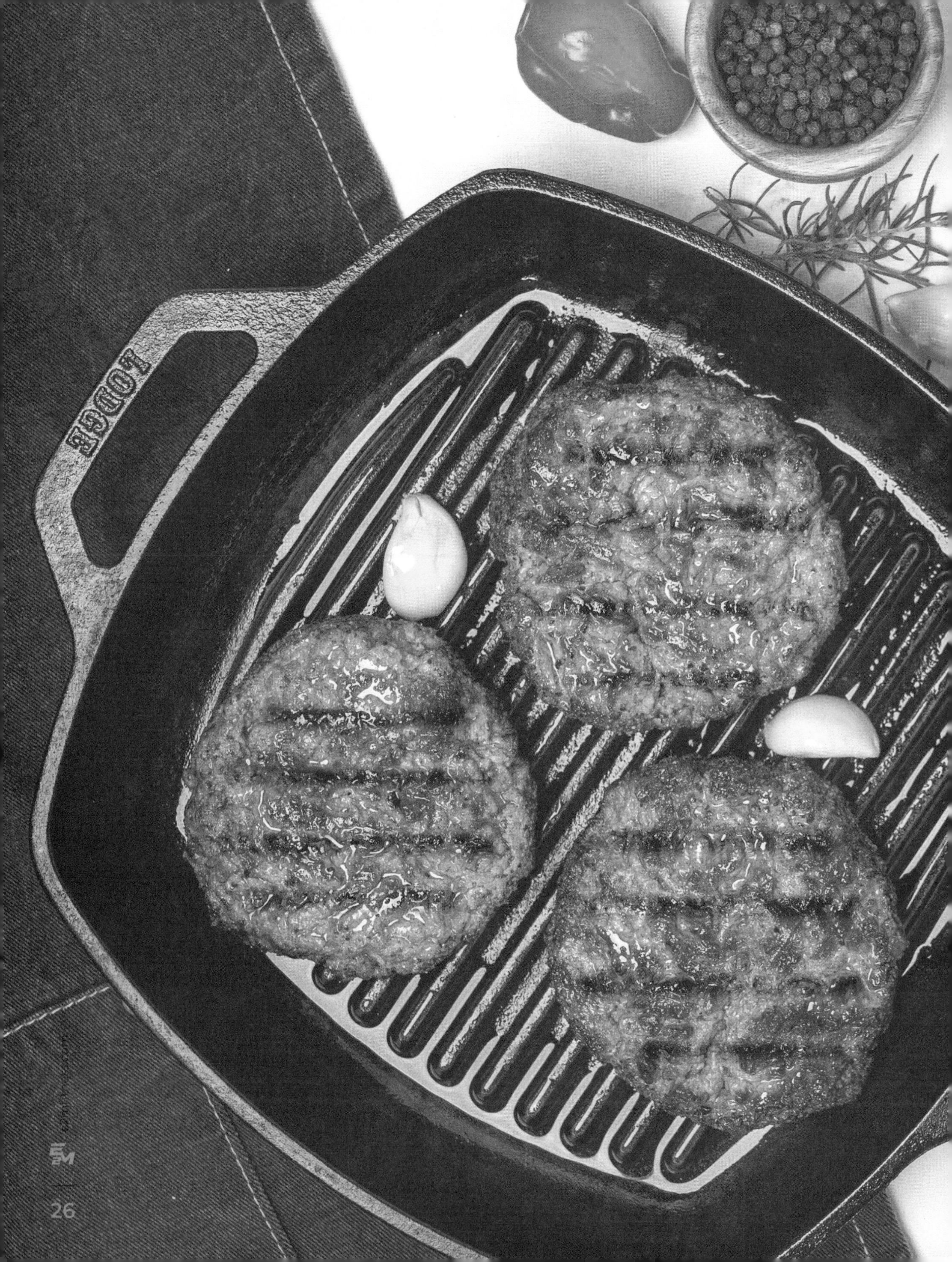
LODGE

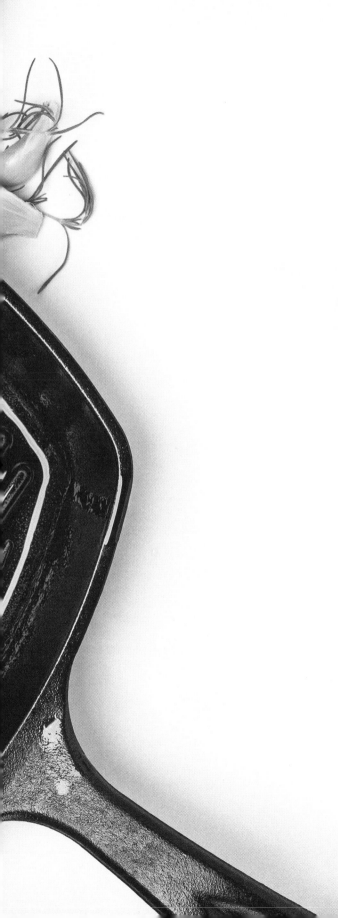

Beef

Beef Taco Wraps
with Chili-Lime Zucchini

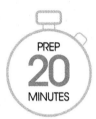

PREP
20
MINUTES

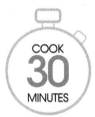

COOK
30
MINUTES

SERVES
4

Chef tip:
The roasted zucchini tastes best when served immediately.

Ingredients

Tacos:

- 2 pounds ground beef (90/10 or leaner)
- ½ cup diced sweet peppers (mini or bell peppers)
- Taco Seasoning (recipe below)
- 3 tablespoons water
- 1 head butter lettuce, leaves separated
- 1 jalapeño, seeded and diced
- 2 avocados, peeled and diced
- 2 tablespoons chopped fresh cilantro

Taco Seasoning:

- 1 tablespoon chili powder
- 1 teaspoon ground cumin
- 1 teaspoon sea salt
- ½ teaspoon ground cayenne pepper
- ½ teaspoon ground garlic

Prep

1. For the Taco Seasoning, whisk together all the ingredients in a small bowl.

Cook

2. Heat a large skillet over medium-high heat; spray with cooking oil. Add the ground beef to the hot pan; cook until browned and almost fully cooked. Add the peppers, and continue to cook until the meat is fully cooked and the peppers are tender. Sprinkle the meat mixture with all of the Taco Seasoning. Drizzle water over the seasoning; stir to combine with the meat.

Chili-Lime Zucchini

- Cooking oil spray
- 5 medium zucchini
- 1 teaspoon olive oil
- 1 tablespoon Chili-Lime Seasoning (see page 106)

Prep

1. To prepare the Chili-Lime Seasoning, combine all the ingredients and mix well; store in an airtight container.

2. Preheat the oven to 425 degrees. Line a baking sheet with parchment paper or spray with cooking oil.

3. Cut the zucchini into 1-inch pieces and put in a bowl. Drizzle olive oil over the zucchini; toss to coat evenly. Sprinkle 1 tablespoon of the Chili-Lime Seasoning over the zucchini; toss until the seasonings are evenly distributed. Spread the zucchini in a single layer on the baking sheet, leaving some space between the pieces.

Cook

4. Bake the zucchini for 5 minutes; flip the pieces and bake for 4 to 7 minutes more, until the zucchini is lightly browned and tender. Overbaking will make the zucchini mushy.

Serve

5. Plate lettuce leaves and spoon the meat mixture into the centers. Top with jalapeño, diced avocado, and fresh cilantro. Serve with Chili-Lime Zucchini for a complete meal.

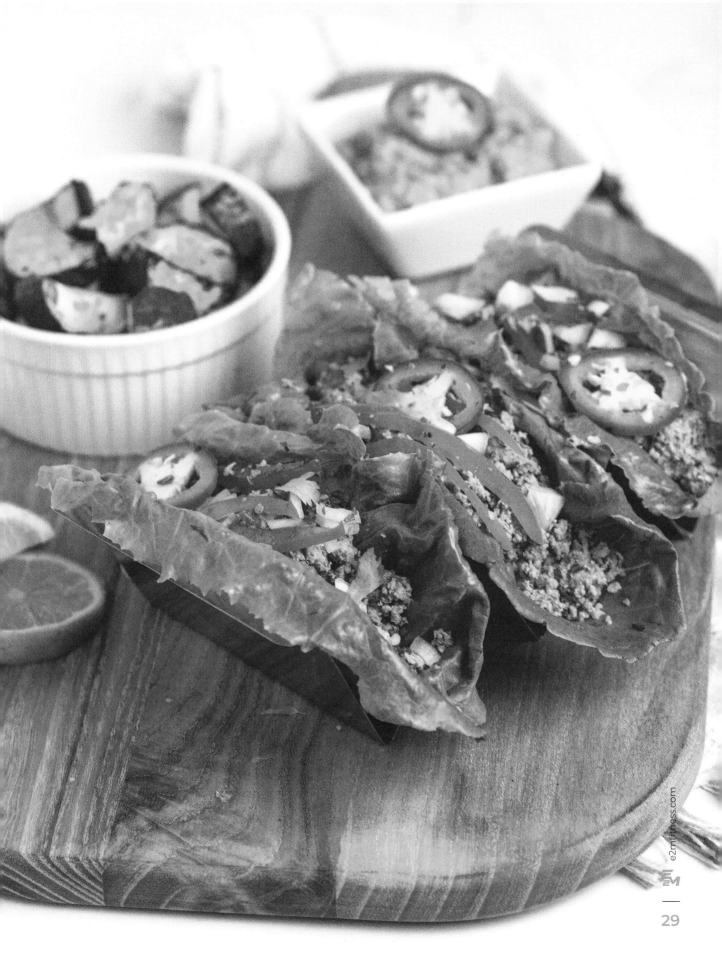

Thai Beef
Zoodles

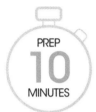

PREP
10
MINUTES

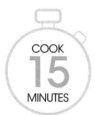

COOK
15
MINUTES

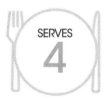

SERVES
4

Ingredients

Beef and Zoodles:

- Cooking oil spray
- 2 pounds ground beef (90/10 or leaner)
- 1 tablespoon Thai Spice Blend (see page 113)
- 1 lime, zest only
- ¼ cup diced bell peppers (red, green, or yellow)

- 2 tablespoons chopped green onions
- ¼ cup shredded carrots
- 2 tablespoons water
- 8 cups zucchini noodles
- 2 tablespoons chopped fresh cilantro

Sauce:

- ¼ cup cashew butter or peanut butter
- 1 lime, juice only

- 1 teaspoon Thai Spice Blend (see page 113)
- ¼ cup water

Prep

1. Combine all the ingredients for the Thai Spice Blend and mix well; store in an airtight container.

2. To make the sauce, combine the cashew butter, lime juice, and 1 teaspoon of the Thai Spice Blend. Add ¼ cup water to thin out the sauce; mix well and taste. If it is not spicy enough, add more seasoning to your liking.

Cook

3. Heat a large skillet over medium-high heat; spray with cooking oil. Add the ground beef, 1 tablespoon of the Thai Spice Blend, and the lime zest; stir frequently, cooking the meat until browned and almost fully cooked. Add the bell peppers, green onions, and shredded carrots; cook for about 2 minutes more, stirring frequently. Stir in 2 tablespoons of water to loosen the spices off the bottom of the pan. Add the zucchini noodles and prepared sauce to the same skillet; sauté for 2 to 4 minutes. Stir thoroughly to combine everything.

Serve

4. Plate the beef, vegetables, and zucchini noodles. Garnish with fresh cilantro.

Cajun Beef
Bowl

Ingredients

Cajun Beef:
- Cooking oil spray
- ½ cup diced red onion
- ½ cup diced bell pepper (any color)
- ¼ cup diced celery
- 2 pounds ground beef (90/10 or leaner)
- 2 tablespoons Cajun Blend (see page 109)

Cauliflower Rice:
- 1 lime, juiced
- 4 cups cauliflower rice, frozen or fresh
- 1 tablespoon Cajun Blend (see page 109)

Toppings (optional):
- 2 avocados, peeled and diced
- ¼ cup chopped fresh parsley
- 1 jalapeño, seeded and diced
- Dash of hot sauce

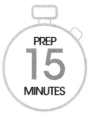

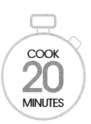

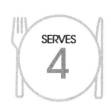

Prep

1. Combine all the ingredients for the Cajun Blend and mix well; store extra in an airtight container.

Cook

2. Heat a large pan or cast-iron skillet over medium heat; spray with cooking oil. Add the red onion, bell pepper, and celery, and cook for 1 minute. Add the ground beef and 2 tablespoons of the Cajun Blend. Stir frequently and cook until the meat is browned and no pink remains; remove the mixture from the pan.

3. In the same pan over medium heat, squeeze the juice from 1 lime; use a wooden spoon to scrape the bottom of the pan to remove any browned beef that remains. This is called fond and adds flavor to the vegetables. Add the frozen cauliflower and 1 tablespoon of the Cajun Blend. Cook for 3 to 4 minutes or until the cauliflower is tender.

Serve

4. Plate the cauliflower rice and top with the Cajun beef mixture. Add optional toppings of avocado, fresh parsley, or diced jalapeño and hot sauce for added heat.

⧎ Success Stories

Josh W., Raleigh, NC

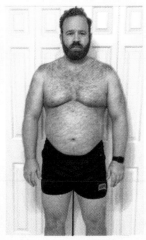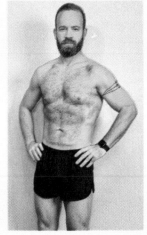

Rounds	Age	Weight Loss
2	41	60

After several Citadel classmates shared their amazing results, I joined E2M fitness while I was navigating being a single parent. After losing weight, getting into the best shape of my life, and meeting an incredible community of people, I've been able to live a life I didn't think was possible—finding a love of hiking, being more active with my kids, and traveling around to E2M meetups whenever I can!

What does the E2M community mean to you?
A genuine family filled with lifelong friends who have encouraged and supported me to live a healthier life.

La'Chandra P., Newton Grove, NC

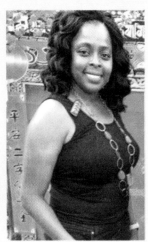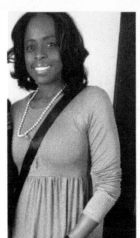

Rounds	Age	Weight Loss
3	47	40

The E2M program has changed my outlook on health and physical fitness. My favorite Bible verse is Philippians 4:13, "I can do ALL things through Christ which strengthened me!"

What does the E2M community mean to you?
The E2M community means so much to me. I love the community because it is so supportive, positive, and uplifting. It's a breath of fresh air in a world that is so divisive.

Non-Scale Victory (NSV)!
My bra size has gone from 40DD to 32DDD—winning!

Asian Beef
Stir-Fry

Ingredients

Beef:

- 1 tablespoon olive oil
- 1 tablespoon Asian Spice Blend (see page 111)
- 2 pounds ground beef (90/10 or leaner)

Vegetables:

- 1 tablespoon olive oil
- ½ head red cabbage, shredded
- ½ head green cabbage, shredded
- 1 cup shredded carrots
- 2 red bell peppers, cut into very thin strips
- 1 cup peanuts, roasted, chopped
- 1½ tablespoons Asian Spice Blend (see page 111)
- 1 or 2 dashes hot sauce
- 2 tablespoons chopped fresh cilantro
- 1 lime (wedges for garnish)

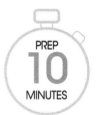

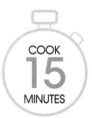

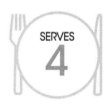

Prep

1. Combine all the ingredients for the Asian Spice Blend and mix well; store in an airtight container.

Cook

2. Heat 1 tablespoon olive oil in a large skillet or wok over medium heat. Add 1 tablespoon of the Asian Spice Blend and stir until fragrant, about 30 seconds. Add the ground beef; cook and stir until browned and no pink remains. Transfer the meat to a plate.

3. To cook the vegetables, heat 1 tablespoon olive oil in the same skillet over medium heat. When the pan is hot and starts to smoke, add the prepared red cabbage, green cabbage, carrots, and red bell pepper strips. Cook for 2 to 3 minutes, stirring occasionally.

4. Add 1½ tablespoons of the Asian Spice Blend. Continue to cook until the vegetables are just tender, an additional 2 to 3 minutes; remove from the heat. Add the hot sauce to the vegetables and mix well.

Serve

5. Plate the slaw mixture and top with the beef; garnish with fresh cilantro, lime wedges, and roasted peanuts.

Zucchini
Boats

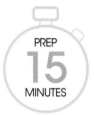

PREP
15
MINUTES

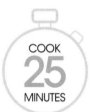

COOK
25
MINUTES

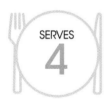

SERVES
4

Ingredients

- 4 large zucchini
- Cooking oil spray
- 1 pound ground beef (90/10 or leaner)
- 1 red onion, diced small
- 1 red bell pepper, diced small
- 1 green bell pepper, diced small
- Fresh cilantro, chopped (for garnish)
- 1½ teaspoons garlic
- 1½ teaspoons smoked paprika
- 1 tablespoon oregano

Prep

1. Slice the zucchini in half vertically, and use a spoon to scoop out the inside of the zucchini. Chop the zucchini flesh and reserve for later. Spray the outside of the zucchini with cooking oil.

2. Preheat the oven to 400 degrees. Line a large baking sheet with parchment paper or spray with cooking oil.

Cook

3. Heat a pan over medium-high heat; spray with cooking oil. Add the ground beef and dry seasonings to the hot pan; cook until browned on both sides and no pink remains. Crumble the meat to roughly the same size as the diced vegetables.

4. Add the diced red onions and bell peppers; cook until tender, 3 to 5 minutes. Combine the meat and vegetables with the reserved zucchini; mix well.

5. Spoon the mixture into the prepped zucchini shells and put them on the baking sheet. Roast in the oven for 20 minutes. Remove from the oven and allow to cool.

Serve

6. Plate two zucchini boats for each serving; top with fresh cilantro.

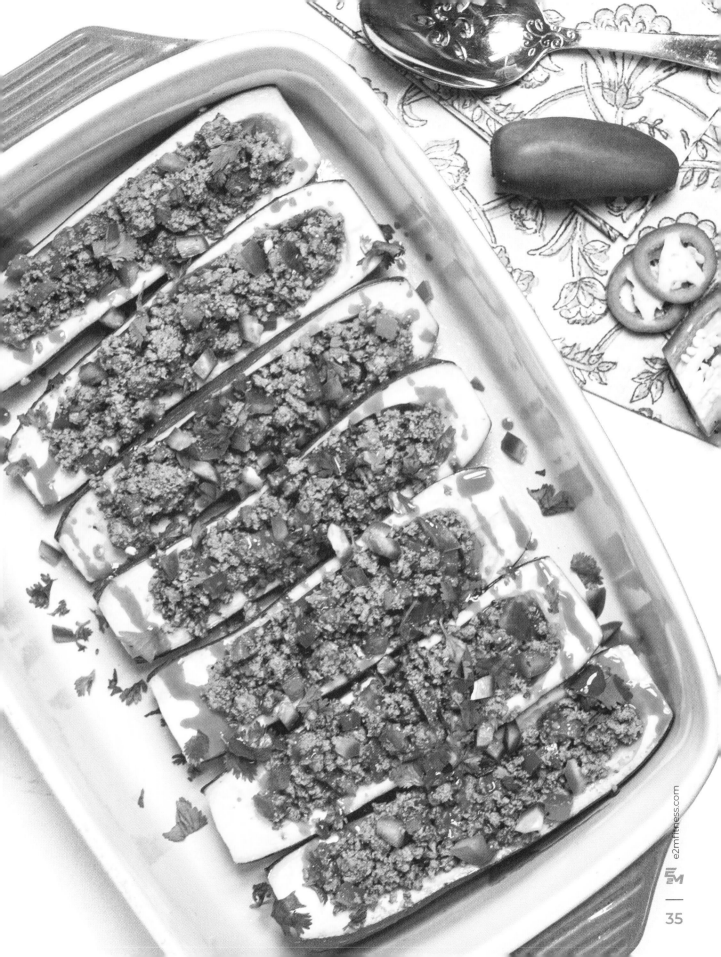

Greek Beef
Bowl

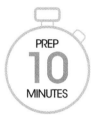

PREP
10
MINUTES

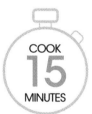

COOK
15
MINUTES

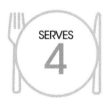

SERVES
4

Ingredients

Vegetables:

- 1 (14-ounce) can artichoke hearts, drained and quartered
- 1 cup sliced black olives
- 1 cup diced English cucumber
- 1 cup diced red bell pepper
- 1 tablespoon olive oil
- 1 lemon, juiced
- ¼ teaspoon sea salt
- ⅛ teaspoon black pepper

Beef:

- Cooking oil spray
- 2 tablespoons Mediterranean Spice Blend (see page 106)
- 2 pounds ground beef (90/10 or leaner)
- Fresh parsley (for garnish)

Prep

1. Combine all the ingredients for the Mediterranean Spice Blend and mix well; store extra in an airtight container.

2. Combine the artichokes, black olives, cucumber, and red bell pepper. Add the olive oil, juice of one lemon, sea salt, and black pepper; toss to combine. Set aside.

Cook

3. Heat a large pan or cast-iron skillet over medium heat; spray with cooking oil. Add 2 tablespoons Mediterranean Spice Blend and stir until fragrant, about 30 seconds. Add the ground beef; cook until browned on both sides and no pink remains.

Serve

4. Plate the vegetable mixture and top with the beef; garnish with fresh parsley.

Baked Cauliflower
Beef Casserole

Ingredients

Beef Base:
- Cooking oil spray
- 1 onion, diced
- 2 celery stalks, diced
- 2 cups diced carrots
- 1 tablespoon ground garlic
- 1½ pounds ground beef (90/10 or leaner)

- 1 tablespoon dried oregano
- 1 tablespoon chopped dried rosemary
- ¼ teaspoon sea salt
- ⅛ teaspoon black pepper

Cauliflower Topping:
- 1 bag frozen cauliflower rice
- 2 tablespoons olive oil
- 1 teaspoon sea salt

- 1 teaspoon black pepper
- 2 tablespoons chopped fresh parsley

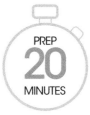

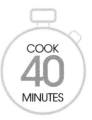

Prep

1. Thaw the frozen cauliflower rice. Preheat the oven to 400 degrees. Spray a casserole dish with cooking oil or line with parchment paper.

Cook

2. For the meat, first heat a large skillet over medium-high heat; spray with cooking oil. Add the onion, celery, and carrots; cook until tender, about 5 minutes. Add the ground meat to the pan and cook until browned. Season with the garlic, oregano, and rosemary. Allow to sauté for 3 to 4 minutes more to develop the flavor.

3. To make the cauliflower topping, combine the thawed cauliflower rice and olive oil; puree with an immersion blender until smooth. Season with the sea salt and black pepper.

4. Spread the meat mixture in the bottom of the prepared casserole dish; top with the cauliflower mixture and smooth with a spoon. Bake for 30 minutes or until the top is brown and bubbly.

Serve

5. Cut the casserole into 4 servings; plate and garnish with fresh parsley.

Korean Beef
Bowl

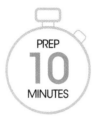

PREP
10
MINUTES

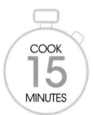

COOK
15
MINUTES

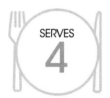

SERVES
4

Ingredients

Base:

- 2 pounds ground beef (90/10 or leaner)
- ½ teaspoon ground garlic
- ½ teaspoon onion powder
- ¼ teaspoon ground ginger
- ¼ teaspoon sea salt
- ⅛ teaspoon crushed red pepper
- Cooking oil spray
- 1 lime, juice and zest
- 4 cups cauliflower rice, frozen or fresh

Toppings:

- 1 cucumber, thinly sliced
- 2 avocados, peeled and diced
- ½ red onion, diced small
- ½ teaspoon sesame seeds
- 1 tablespoon thinly sliced green onions

Prep

1. Combine the ground beef, garlic, onion powder, ginger, sea salt, and crushed red pepper; mix thoroughly.

Cook

2. Heat a pan over medium-high heat; spray with cooking oil. Add the seasoned meat to the hot pan; cook until browned on both sides and no pink remains. Transfer the cooked meat to a plate.

3. Turn the heat down to medium. Squeeze the juice from ½ lime into the pan; use a wooden spoon to remove the cooked-on meat from the bottom of the pan and stir. Add the cauliflower rice; sauté for 5 to 8 minutes.

Serve

4. Plate the cauliflower rice as the base followed by the seasoned beef; add the prepared cucumber, avocado, and red onion. Garnish with sesame seeds, lime zest, and juice from the remaining ½ lime.

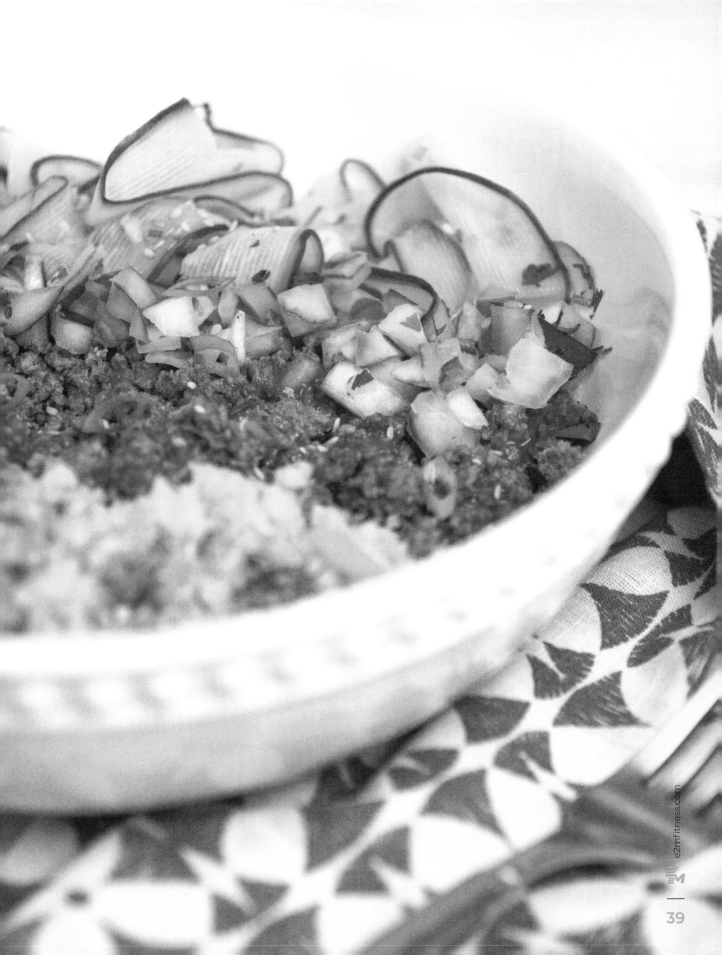

Peppered Beef
and Broccoli

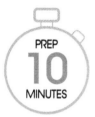

PREP
10
MINUTES

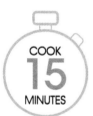

COOK
15
MINUTES

SERVES
4

Ingredients

- 1 teaspoon ground garlic
- ½ teaspoon ground ginger
- ¼ teaspoon sea salt
- ⅛ teaspoon crushed red pepper
- ⅛ teaspoon black pepper
- 2 tablespoons Dijon mustard
- 2 tablespoons rice vinegar, divided
- 8 cups broccoli florets

- 2 pounds ground beef (90/10 or leaner)
- Cooking oil spray
- 2 avocados, peeled and sliced
- Sesame seeds (for garnish)
- Hot sauce (optional for garnish)
- 4 cups cooked cauliflower rice (serving option)

Prep

1. Combine the garlic, ginger, sea salt, crushed red pepper, black pepper, Dijon mustard, and 1 tablespoon of the rice vinegar. Mix thoroughly. Add the ground beef to the marinade and combine.

Cook

2. Heat a pan over medium-high heat; spray with cooking oil. Add the seasoned meat to the hot pan; cook until browned on both sides and no pink remains. Remove from the pan.

3. Pour the remaining 1 tablespoon of rice vinegar into the pan; use a wooden spoon to scrape the bottom of the pan to remove any cooked-on meat. This step adds additional flavor to the broccoli. Add broccoli to the pan and sauté for 3 to 5 minutes or until the broccoli has turned bright green.

Serve

4. Plate the beef and broccoli with ½ avocado for each serving; garnish with sesame seeds and hot sauce, if preferred. This meal is delicious served over cauliflower rice.

Taco
Salad

Ingredients

Taco Meat:
- 2 pounds ground beef (90/10 or leaner)
- 1 teaspoon sea salt
- ½ teaspoon ground garlic
- ½ teaspoon paprika
- ½ teaspoon ground cumin
- ½ teaspoon chili powder
- 1 teaspoon lime zest
- Cooking oil spray

Salad:
- 8 cups chopped mixed greens
- 1 cup chopped red bell pepper
- ½ cup diced red onion
- 1 cup diced cucumber
- 2 avocados, peeled and diced
- 1 tablespoon chopped fresh cilantro

Prep

1. Put the ground meat into a bowl; add the sea salt, garlic, paprika, cumin, chili powder, and lime zest. Mix thoroughly.

Cook

2. Heat a pan over medium-high heat; spray with cooking oil. Add the ground beef to the hot pan; cook until browned on both sides and no pink remains.

Serve

3. Plate the mixed greens; add the cooked meat. Top with red bell pepper, red onion, cucumber, and avocado. Garnish with fresh cilantro.

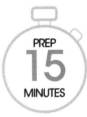

PREP
15
MINUTES

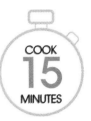

COOK
15
MINUTES

SERVES
4

Garlic and Herb Burger
Lettuce Wrap with Carrot Fries

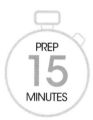

PREP
15
MINUTES

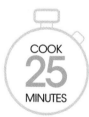

COOK
25
MINUTES

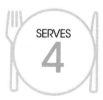

SERVES
4

Ingredients

Burgers:
- 2 pounds ground beef (90/10 or leaner)
- 1½ tablespoons ground garlic
- 1½ teaspoons chopped fresh thyme
- 1½ teaspoons finely chopped fresh chives
- 1 teaspoon sea salt
- 1 teaspoon black pepper
- ½ teaspoon crushed red pepper
- ½ teaspoon ground mustard
- Cooking oil spray
- 1 head iceberg lettuce, leaves

Carrot Fries:
- 8 cups baby carrots
- 1½ tablespoons chopped fresh parsley
- 1½ tablespoons paprika
- 1½ tablespoons olive oil
- 2 teaspoons sea salt
- 2 teaspoons black pepper
- 1½ teaspoons dried thyme

Optional Toppings:
- Avocado slices; sautéed mushrooms or peppers

Prep

1. Preheat the oven to 425 degrees. Line a baking sheet with parchment paper or spray with cooking oil for the carrot fries.

2. To prepare the burgers, combine the ground beef, garlic, thyme, chives, sea salt, black pepper, crushed red pepper, and ground mustard; mix well. Form 4 to 6 patties and press a thumbprint into the center of each patty to prevent the burger from shrinking in size during the cooking process.

3. In a separate bowl, prepare the carrot fries by combining the baby carrots with the parsley, paprika, olive oil, sea salt, black pepper, and thyme. Spread out the carrots in single layer on the baking sheet.

Cook

4. Bake the carrots for 20 to 25 minutes, flipping halfway through.

5. While the carrots are baking, heat a large skillet over medium-high heat; spray with cooking oil. Cook the patties for 5 to 8 minutes per side, until the internal temperature reaches 160 degrees or your desired doneness.

Serve

6. Use the iceberg lettuce leaves as the bun for the burgers; add optional toppings such as avocado slices, sautéed mushrooms, or sautéed sweet peppers, if desired. Serve with carrot fries.

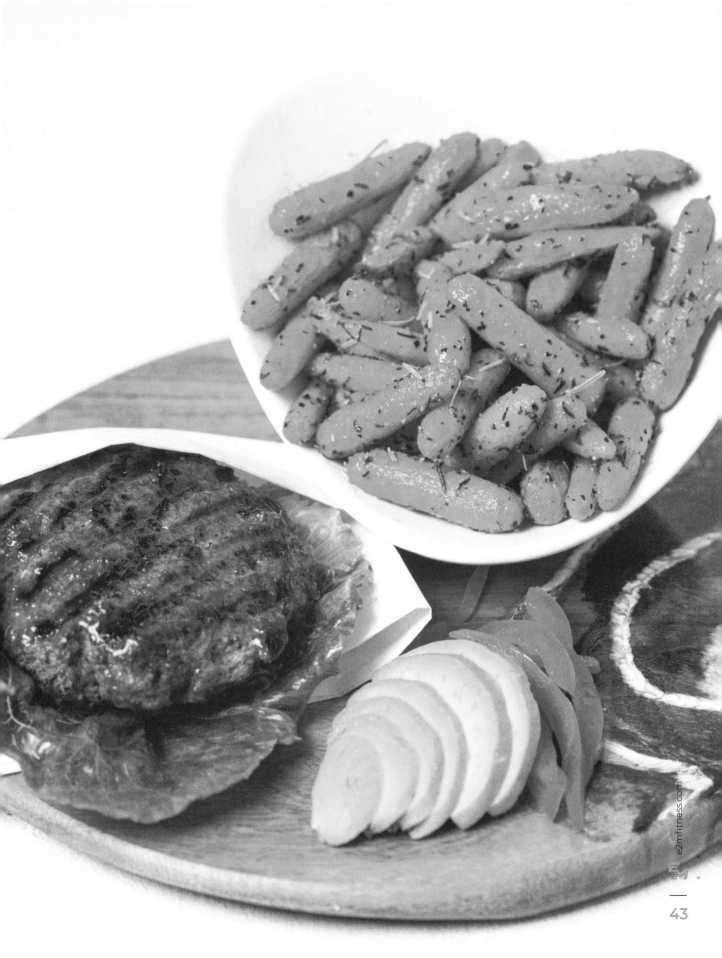

Christy M., Princeton, NC

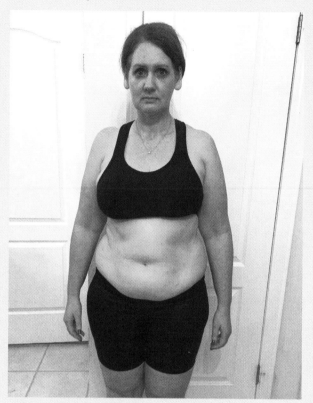
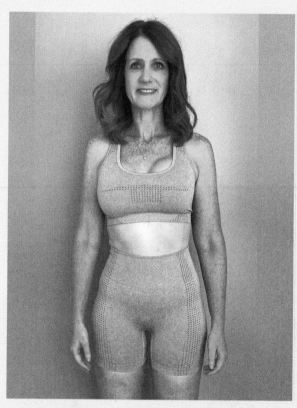

Rounds	Age	Weight Loss
3	47	54

I wanted to be engaged in life and not watch it pass me by. I wanted to do things and wear certain clothes. Now I get to go places, do things, and wear smaller size clothes.

What were you hoping to gain from your E2M experience?
After my husband's near heart attack and heart surgery, I knew we needed a change. We were introduced to E2M fitness shortly after that and I have never regretted my decision to join this lifestyle. Now we're active and adventurous! We hike, bicycle, paraglide, snorkel, cliff dive, etc.!

Beef Burrito
Bowl

Ingredients

Guacamole:
- 2 avocados, peeled and diced
- 2 tablespoons chopped fresh cilantro
- ¼ cup diced red onion
- 1 lime, juiced
- ¼ teaspoon sea salt
- ⅛ teaspoon black pepper

Cauliflower Rice:
- 1 tablespoon olive oil
- 2 (12-ounce) bags cauliflower rice, frozen or shelf stable
- 1 lime, juiced
- 1 tablespoon chopped fresh cilantro
- ¼ teaspoon sea salt
- ⅛ teaspoon black pepper

Meat Filling:
- Cooking oil spray
- ½ cup diced red onion
- 1 jalapeño, seeded and minced
- 1½ pounds ground beef (90/10 or leaner)
- 1½ tablespoons Burrito Seasoning (recipe below)

Burrito Seasoning:
- ½ teaspoon sea salt
- 1 teaspoon ground garlic
- 1 teaspoon paprika
- 1 teaspoon ground cumin
- 1 teaspoon chili powder
- 1 lime, zested

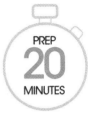

PREP
20
MINUTES

COOK
30
MINUTES

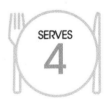

SERVES
4

Prep

1. For the Burrito Seasoning, whisk together all the ingredients; store in an airtight container.

2. To make the guacamole, combine the avocado, cilantro, red onion, lime juice, sea salt, and black pepper; mix well. Cover tightly and refrigerate.

Cook

3. For the meat, first heat a large nonstick skillet over medium heat; spray with cooking oil. Add the red onions and jalapeño; cook until tender, 3 to 4 minutes, stirring frequently. Add the ground beef and 1½ tablespoons of the Burrito Seasoning. Cook until the meat is browned on both sides and no pink remains. Remove from the heat and set aside.

4. For the cauliflower rice, heat a nonstick skillet over medium heat and pour in the olive oil. Add the cauliflower rice and cook for 3 to 4 minutes, until the cauliflower is heated and fully cooked. Add the lime juice and cilantro; season with sea salt and black pepper to taste.

Serve

5. Layer the burrito bowls with cauliflower rice as the base; top with seasoned ground beef and vegetables, then guacamole.

Beef Stuffed
Peppers

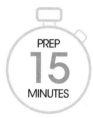

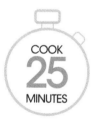

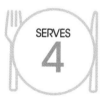

Ingredients

- Cooking oil spray
- 4 large bell peppers (any color)
- ¼ teaspoon sea salt
- 2 tablespoons olive oil
- 1 red onion, diced
- 3 garlic cloves, minced
- 1½ pounds ground beef (90/10 or leaner)
- 1½ teaspoons chili powder
- 1 teaspoon sea salt
- ½ teaspoon ground cumin
- ¼ teaspoon dried oregano
- 1 (12-ounce) bag cauliflower rice (frozen or shelf stable)
- Fresh parsley, chopped (for garnish)

Prep

1. Preheat the oven to 425 degrees. Spray a baking dish with cooking oil.

2. Cut the bell peppers in half from stem to bottom; remove the seeds and core. Put the peppers (cut-side up) in a baking dish. Spray the peppers with cooking oil and sprinkle with ¼ teaspoon sea salt.

Cook

3. Bake the peppers for 15 minutes, until lightly browned. Remove from the oven and set aside. The oven will be used later at 425 degrees.

4. Heat a large nonstick skillet over medium heat; pour in the olive oil. Add the red onions; stir frequently and cook until soft, 3 to 4 minutes. Add the garlic and cook for 1 minute more. Add the ground beef, chili powder, sea salt, cumin, and oregano. Cook for 4 to 5 minutes, breaking the meat up with a spoon until the meat is browned and no pink remains. Add the cauliflower rice and stir to combine.

5. Spoon the meat filling evenly into the peppers; return the filled peppers to the oven for 5 minutes at 425 degrees.

Serve

6. Plate the stuffed peppers; garnish with fresh parsley.

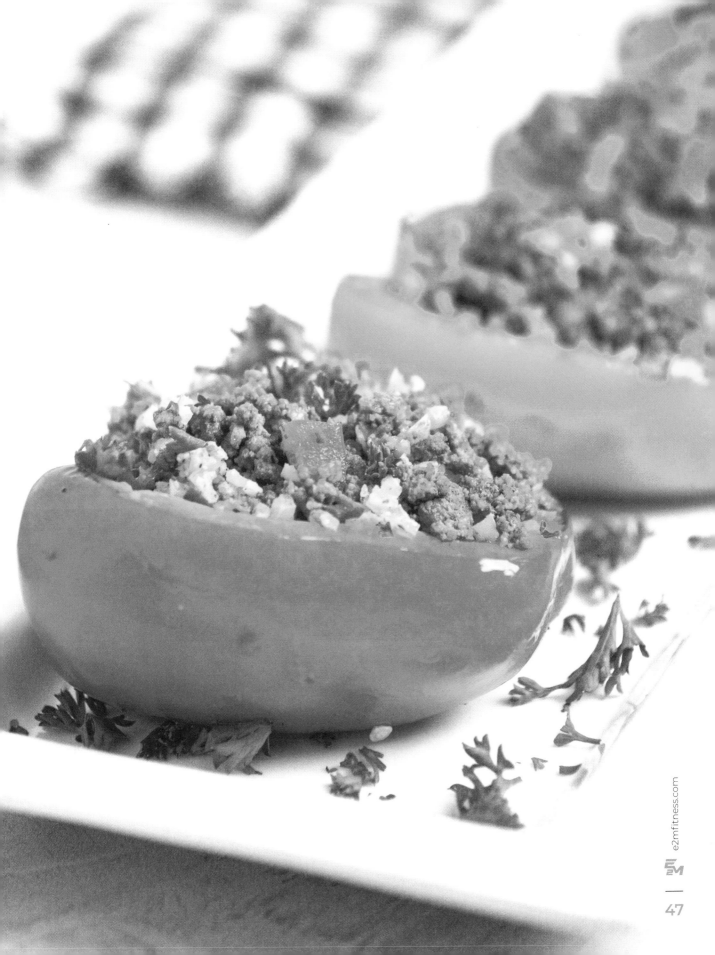

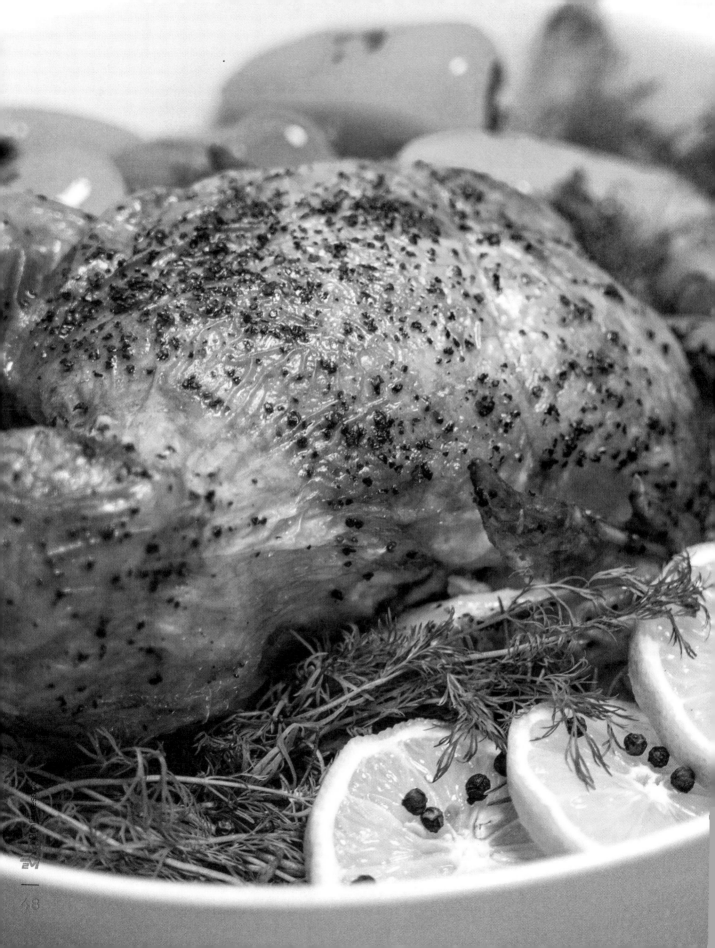

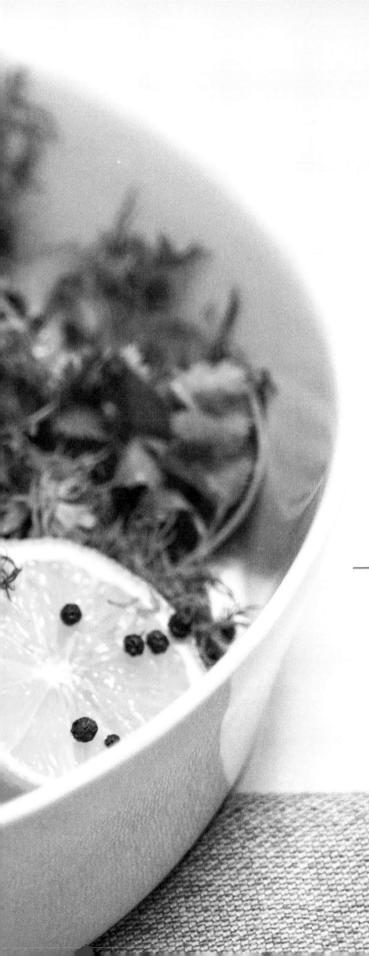

Poultry

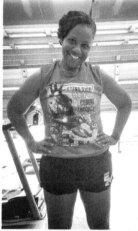 Success Stories

Sudie H., Summerville, SC

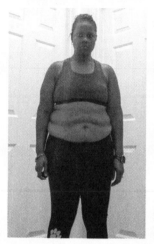 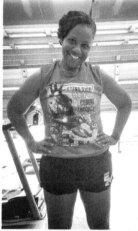

Rounds	Age	Weight Loss
12	42	100

I'm known on the E2M fitness page as the "drip queen" or the #OperationActUp cheerleader. I'm a wife, minister, and project manager. I just love to inspire people to simply make it look excellent. SMILE.

How has E2M fitness changed your life?
I'm now always aware of what I'm eating and how it's affecting my body. No more hypertension medication!

Non-Scale Victory (NSV)!
I went from wearing size 14 to size 8 dresses. I decreased my 5K time by five minutes and acquired new 5K and 10K personal records.

Allie B., Irmo, SC

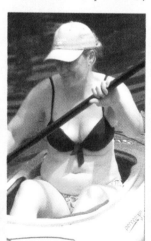 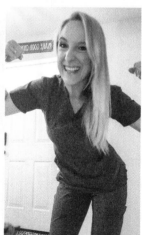

Rounds	Age	Weight Loss
6	41	25

I'm a mom of three, ER nurse turned DNP, and am now in primary care. I started E2M fitness to get ready for my wedding, and it changed into more. I wanted to represent health if I was going to be telling my patients they needed to get healthy.

What is your biggest E2M fitness accomplishment?
I thought it was the confidence I had on my wedding and graduation day, but truly, it's the people I bring in with me. I enjoy watching their excitement when they hit goal after goal.

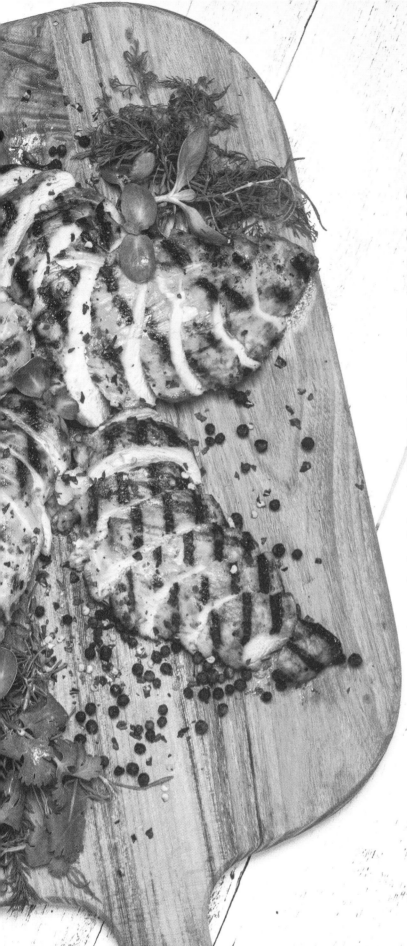

Turkey

Citrus Herb Roasted
Turkey and Brussels Sprouts

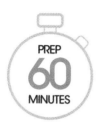

PREP
60
MINUTES

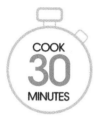

COOK
30
MINUTES

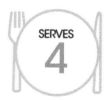

SERVES
4

Meal prep idea:

Prepare the turkey and vegetables, let cool, and divide into airtight containers. Store in the refrigerator for up to three days.

Note:

This complete meal is an excellent dish for entertaining large groups.

Ingredients

Citrus and Herb Roasted Turkey:

- 1 orange, zested and juiced
- 1 lemon, zested and juiced
- 2 sprigs fresh thyme, chopped
- 2 sprigs fresh rosemary, chopped
- 3 sage leaves, chopped
- 1½ teaspoons sea salt
- 1 teaspoon black pepper
- 1 teaspoon ground garlic
- 1 tablespoon olive oil
- 3 pounds turkey breast

Brussels Sprouts:

- 2 tablespoons olive oil
- ⅛ teaspoon black pepper
- 8 cups of brussels sprouts, quartered
- 1 tablespoon Dijon mustard
- ¼ teaspoon sea salt
- 1 tablespoon vinegar
- 4 apples, cored, diced
- 1 cup pitted and quartered fresh cherries
- 1 tablespoon dried thyme
- 1 cup slivered almonds

Prep

1. In a large mixing bowl, combine the orange zest and juice, lemon zest and juice, thyme, rosemary, sage, sea salt, black pepper, garlic, and olive oil. Add the turkey breast and coat until completely covered, rubbing the marinade into the skin. Refrigerate and allow to marinate for at least 1 hour.

2. Line a rimmed baking sheet with parchment paper or spray with cooking oil. Preheat the oven to 350 degrees. Put the turkey on the prepared baking sheet; pour the remaining marinade over the turkey.

Cook

3. Bake the turkey breast for 25 to 30 minutes, depending on the size. Make sure that the internal temperature reaches 165 degrees before removing it from the oven.

4. In a large ovenproof cast-iron skillet, heat the olive oil over medium-high heat. Toss the brussels sprouts in Dijon mustard, sea salt, and black pepper. Cook for 15 to 20 minutes, stirring frequently. Add the vinegar and stir to remove any cooked-on bits from the bottom of the pan. Add the diced apples, cherries, and thyme; cook for another 3 minutes and remove from the heat.

Serve

5. Plate the brussels sprouts and apple mixture on a platter; top with the roasted turkey. Garnish with slivered almonds.

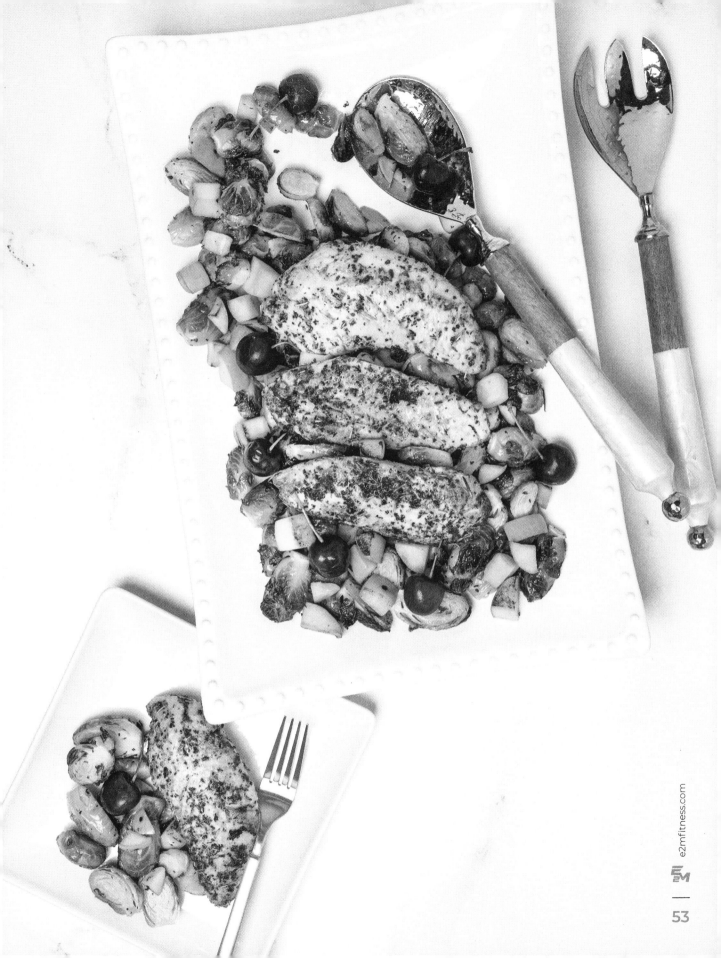

Curry Turkey
Bowl

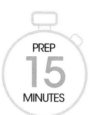

PREP
15
MINUTES

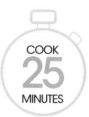

COOK
25
MINUTES

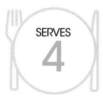

SERVES
4

Ingredients

- Cooking oil spray
- 1 medium onion, chopped
- 2 tablespoons curry powder
- 1½ teaspoons ground garlic
- ¼ teaspoon ground ginger
- ¼ teaspoon ground cumin
- ⅛ teaspoon ground cayenne pepper
- 2 pounds diced turkey breast
- 2 cups of water
- 4 cups cauliflower rice, frozen or shelf stable, prepared
- ½ cup chopped fresh cilantro, divided
- 2 limes, zested and juiced
- ½ teaspoon sea salt

Cook

1. Spray oil in the bottom of a dutch oven or deep pot, and heat over medium heat; add the onion and cook until transparent, 2 to 3 minutes. Add the curry, garlic, ginger, cumin, and cayenne; heat until you start to smell the spices, being careful not to burn them. This is called "blooming" the spices and is a technique used in many cultures. Add the diced turkey to the pot; stir to coat in spices.

2. Pour 2 cups of water in the pot; the water needs to cover the turkey. Stir and cook the turkey for 20 minutes, or until the internal temperature reaches 165 degrees. Turn off the heat and allow to cool.

3. Follow package directions for heating the cauliflower rice you prefer; add ¼ cup of the cilantro and the juice and zest of 1 lime. Toss to combine and set aside.

Serve

4. Plate the cauliflower rice and top with curried turkey. Garnish with fresh lime juice and zest and the remaining ¼ cup cilantro.

Korean Turkey
Bowl

Ingredients

Turkey:

- 2 pounds ground turkey
- ½ teaspoon ground garlic
- ½ teaspoon onion powder
- ¼ teaspoon ground ginger
- ¼ teaspoon sea salt
- ⅛ teaspoon black pepper
- ⅛ teaspoon crushed red pepper
- Cooking oil spray

Cauliflower and Toppings:

- 2 limes, zested and juiced
- 4 cups cauliflower rice, frozen or fresh, prepared
- 1 cucumber, thinly sliced
- ½ red onion, diced small
- 2 avocados, peeled and diced
- ½ teaspoon sesame seeds

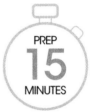

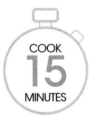

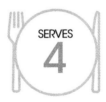

Prep

1. Combine the ground turkey in a bowl with the garlic, onion powder, ginger, sea salt, black pepper, and crushed red pepper. Mix thoroughly.

Cook

2. Heat a pan over medium-high heat; spray with cooking oil. Add the seasoned meat to the hot pan; cook until browned on both sides and no pink remains. Transfer the cooked meat to a plate.

3. Turn the heat down to medium heat, squeeze the juice of ½ lime into the pan; use a wooden spoon to remove the cooked-on meat from the bottom of the pan and stir. Add the cauliflower rice to the pan; sauté for 5 to 8 minutes.

Serve

4. Plate the cauliflower rice; top with ground turkey. Add the cucumber, red onion, and avocado. Garnish with sesame seeds and the remaining lime zest and lime juice as preferred.

E2M Success Stories

Mandy & Brandon P., Moncks Corner, SC

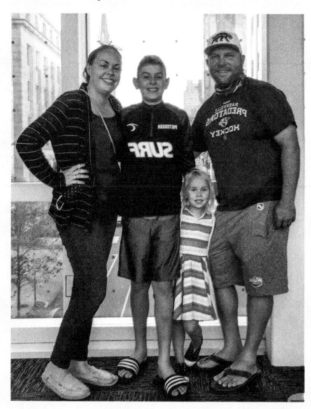 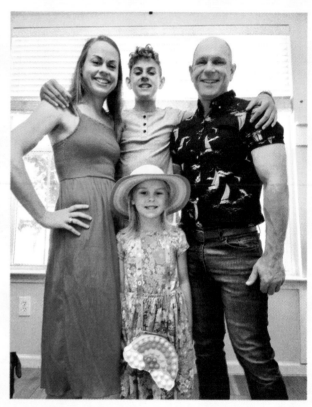

Rounds	Age	Weight Loss
2	38, 39	50

What does the E2M community mean to you?
The E2M community is a safe place where people come together to support each other, no matter where they are on their fitness journey!

How has E2M fitness changed your life?
E2M fitness taught us how to eat food that fuels our body and has given us the tools to show our children what a sustainable, active, and healthy lifestyle looks like. We are forever grateful!

Spicy Turkey
Zoodle Bowl

Ingredients

Turkey and Zoodles:

- 2 pounds ground turkey
- 1½ teaspoons smoked paprika
- ½ teaspoon chili powder
- ¼ teaspoon sea salt
- ⅛ teaspoon black pepper
- 2 tablespoons olive oil
- 1 cup diced red bell peppers
- 1 cup shredded carrots
- 8 cups zucchini noodles
- 2 tablespoons chopped fresh cilantro
- 1 lime, zested
- ½ teaspoon red pepper flakes

Cashew Sauce:

- ¼ cup cashew butter or peanut butter
- 1 lime, juiced and zested
- 3 tablespoons water

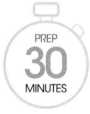

PREP
30
MINUTES

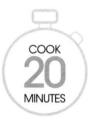

COOK
20
MINUTES

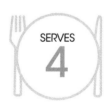

SERVES
4

Prep

1. In a bowl, combine the ground turkey, smoked paprika, chili powder, sea salt, and black pepper; mix thoroughly. Refrigerate for 30 minutes.

2. To make the cashew sauce, combine the cashew butter, lime juice, and add the water to thin out the sauce.

Cook

3. Heat the olive oil in a large pan over medium heat. Add the bell peppers and carrots; cook for about 2 minutes, stirring frequently until vegetables are tender. Stir in some water to loosen the spices off the bottom of the pan. Add the seasoned meat to the hot pan with the vegetable mixture; cook until the meat is browned on both sides and no pink remains, 10 to 12 minutes. Transfer to a plate.

4. Keep the pan at medium heat; add the zucchini noodles and cashew sauce. Sauté for 2 to 4 minutes, stirring to combine.

Serve

5. Plate the zucchini noodles, and top with the turkey-vegetable mixture. Garnish with fresh cilantro and lime zest.

Roasted Cabbage
and Turkey Stacks

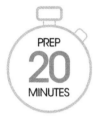

PREP
20
MINUTES

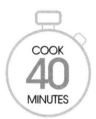

COOK
40
MINUTES

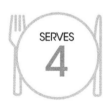

SERVES
4

Ingredients

Cabbage Steaks:
- 1 head red or green cabbage
- Cooking oil spray
- 1 tablespoon smoked paprika
- 1½ teaspoons ground garlic
- ¼ teaspoon sea salt
- ⅛ teaspoon black pepper

Turkey:
- 2 pounds ground turkey
- ½ teaspoon ground garlic
- ½ teaspoon dried thyme
- ½ teaspoon chili powder
- 1 cup apple, diced small

Garnish:
- 2 avocados, peeled and diced
- ¼ cup chopped fresh cilantro
- 1 lime, zested and juiced

Prep

1. Preheat the oven to 400 degrees. Line a baking sheet with parchment paper or spray with cooking oil.

2. Slice the cabbage into ½-inch-thick rounds, like steaks; these will form the base of the dish. Spray each side with oil and sprinkle with the paprika, garlic, sea salt, and black pepper; arrange on the baking sheet, cutting rounds in half if needed.

Cook

3. Roast the cabbage steaks in the oven for 25 to 30 minutes, or until the cabbage is tender.

4. Heat a large skillet over medium heat; spray with cooking oil. Add the ground meat to the hot pan and sprinkle with the garlic, thyme, and chili powder. Cook for 10 to 15 minutes until browned on both sides and almost fully cooked. Add the diced apple and cook until tender.

Serve

5. Plate the cabbage steaks; top with ground turkey and apples.
   Optional: Garnish with diced avocado, fresh cilantro, lime zest, and lime juice.

Meal prep idea:
Prepare the ground meat and let cool, then divide into airtight containers. Store the roasted cabbage separately in a gallon plastic bag or airtight container. Keep in the refrigerator for up to three days.

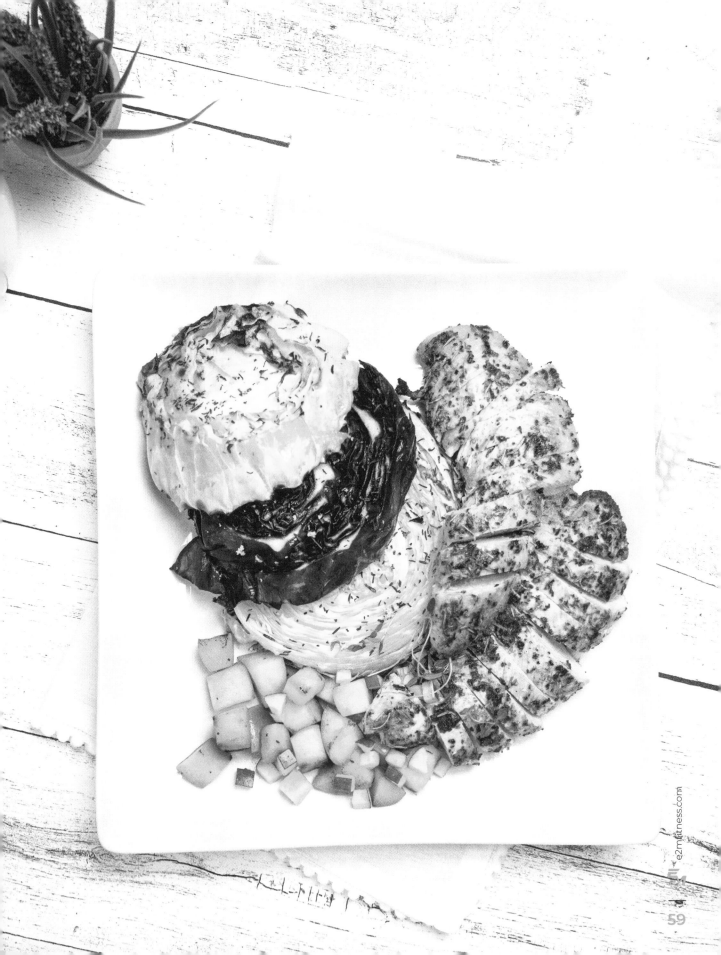

Greek Turkey
Bowl

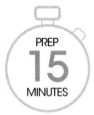

PREP
15
MINUTES

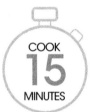

COOK
15
MINUTES

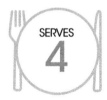

SERVES
4

Ingredients

Vegetables:
- 4 cups shredded cabbage
- 4 cups spinach
- 1 cup diced red bell peppers
- 1 lime, juiced

- ¼ cup chopped fresh cilantro
- 1 cup sliced black olives
- ¼ teaspoon sea salt
- ⅛ teaspoon black pepper

Turkey:
- 1 tablespoon olive oil
- 1 teaspoon dried rosemary
- 1 teaspoon dried oregano

- 1½ teaspoons ground garlic
- 2 pounds ground turkey
- Fresh parsley (for garnish)

Prep

1. Combine the cabbage, spinach, black olives, and red bell pepper. Add the juice of 1 lime with the cilantro, sea salt, and black pepper; toss to combine.

Cook

2. Heat 1 tablespoon olive oil in a large skillet or wok over medium heat. Add the dried rosemary, oregano, and garlic; stir until fragrant, about 30 seconds. Add the ground turkey; cook and stir until browned and no pink remains.

Serve

3. Plate the vegetable mixture and top with turkey; garnish with parsley.

Low-Carb Turkey Burgers
with Zucchini Fries

Ingredients

Turkey Burgers:
- 2 pounds ground turkey
- 1½ tablespoons ground garlic
- 1 tablespoon smoked paprika
- 1 teaspoon chili powder
- 1 teaspoon sea salt
- 1 teaspoon black pepper
- ½ teaspoon ground mustard
- Cooking oil spray
- 1 head iceberg lettuce
- ½ cup chia seeds

Optional Toppings:
- 1 onion, thinly sliced
- 2 cups diced bella mushrooms
- 2 avocados, peeled and sliced

Prep

1. Combine the ground turkey, chia seeds, garlic, smoked paprika, chili powder, sea salt, black pepper, and ground mustard; mix thoroughly. Form 4 to 6 patties from the mixture, and press a thumbprint into the center of each patty to prevent the burger from shrinking in size during the cooking process.

Cook

2. Heat a large skillet over medium-high heat; spray with cooking oil. Add the patties and cook for 5 to 8 minutes per side, until the internal temperature reaches 165 degrees or your desired doneness. Remove from pan.

3. Keep the pan at medium-high heat; add the onions and mushrooms. Sauté for 5 to 10 minutes, or until tender.

Serve

Use the iceberg lettuce leaves as the bun; add the avocado slices, sautéed onions, or sautéed mushrooms. Serve with zucchini fries.

Zucchini Fries:
- 8 cups sliced zucchini
- 1½ tablespoons olive oil
- 1½ tablespoons chopped fresh parsley
- 1½ tablespoons paprika
- 1½ teaspoons dried thyme
- 2 teaspoons sea salt
- 2 teaspoons black pepper

Prep

1. Preheat the oven to 425 degrees. Line a baking sheet with parchment paper.

2. Combine the zucchini slices in a large bowl with the olive oil, parsley, paprika, thyme, sea salt, and black pepper. Toss to coat evenly.

Cook

3. Arrange the zucchini in a single layer on the baking sheet. Bake for 20 to 25 minutes, flipping halfway through. Remove from the oven; sprinkle additional sea salt over the zucchini fries while still hot.

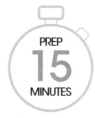

PREP
15
MINUTES

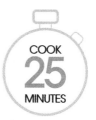

COOK
25
MINUTES

SERVES
4

⧓ Success Stories

Cameron T., Moseley, VA

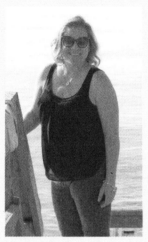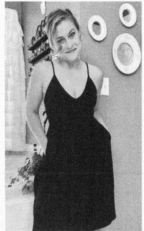

Rounds	Age	Weight Loss
12	47	60

E2M fitness is my absolute daily medicine. I'm the wife of an army retiree and mom to six children and one grandbaby. Busy and chaos go hand in hand in our home! The E2M program allows me to get my stuff done when I can, and still commit to others to support and be supported. I call that a WIN-WIN! When illness crept in, I fought my way through fatigue and a severely compromised immune system. There's no doubt that had I not built myself up prior to my illness, my outcome would have been sorely different.

Non-Scale Victory (NSV)!
I'm tougher physically and mentally than I've ever been!

Marissa S., Fredonia, NY

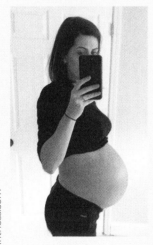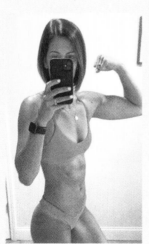

Rounds	Age	Weight Loss
10	35	10

I joined E2M fitness to improve my overall health after having my second child. The program helped me to achieve my goal physique, and I've gained many positive relationships and friendships. I've also learned to see food as fuel and how to eat foods that will support my fitness journey.

What is your favorite type of workout?
Strength training.

What does the E2M community mean to you?
E2M has provided me with a positive and healthy lifestyle filled with unwavering support from a family of like-minded people.

Mediterranean Turkey
Meatball and Vegetable Skewers

Ingredients

Vegetables:
- 2 red bell peppers, diced in large pieces
- 2 green bell peppers, diced in large pieces
- 1 (14-ounce) can artichoke hearts, drained
- 1 (6-ounce) can whole black olives, drained
- 1 tablespoon chopped fresh parsley (for garnish)
- 1 lemon, zested and juiced (for garnish)

Greek Herb Marinade:
- 2 tablespoons chopped fresh parsley
- 2 tablespoons olive oil
- 1 tablespoon paprika
- 1 tablespoon Dijon mustard
- 1 tablespoon apple cider vinegar
- 1½ teaspoons dried oregano

Meatballs:
- 10 wooden skewers
- 2 pounds ground turkey
- ¼ cup chia seeds
- 2 teaspoons ground garlic
- 2 teaspoons Herbs de Provence seasoning (see page 107)
- ¼ teaspoon sea salt
- ⅛ teaspoon black pepper
- Cooking oil spray

- 1½ teaspoons dried basil
- 1 teaspoon ground garlic
- 1 lemon, zested and juiced
- ¼ teaspoon sea salt
- ⅛ teaspoon black pepper

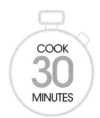

PREP
30
MINUTES

COOK
30
MINUTES

SERVES
4

Prep

1. Soak the wooden skewers in water for 30 minutes prior to using, in order to prevent splintering and burning.

2. Prepare the Greek herb marinade in a large bowl by combining all the ingredients; mix thoroughly. Add the prepared vegetables to the marinade and refrigerate while preparing the meatballs.

3. To prepare the meatballs, combine the ground turkey, chia seeds, garlic, Italian seasoning, sea salt, and black pepper; mix thoroughly. Refrigerate for 30 minutes.

4. Preheat the oven to 400 degrees. Line two baking sheets with parchment paper or spray with cooking oil.

5. Remove the meat mixture from the refrigerator; form the meat mixture into 1-inch balls, and arrange on one of the prepared sheet pans.

Cook

6. Bake the meatballs for 15 to 20 minutes, or until meatballs are browned and cooked through.

7. Thread the red bell peppers, green bell peppers, artichoke hearts, and whole olives on skewers, alternating the pieces. Put the skewers on the other prepared sheet pan and add to the oven. Bake for 8 to 10 minutes.

Serve

8. Plate the meatballs with the vegetable skewers, and garnish with fresh parsley, lemon juice, and lemon zest.

Mandarin Turkey
Stir-Fry

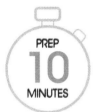

PREP
10
MINUTES

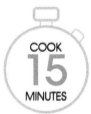

COOK
15
MINUTES

SERVES
4

Ingredients

Turkey:
- 1 tablespoon olive oil
- 2 pounds ground turkey
- 1 tablespoon spice blend (recipe below)

Spice Blend:
- 1 tablespoon dried cilantro
- 1 teaspoon dried basil
- 1 teaspoon onion powder
- 1 teaspoon crushed red pepper
- ¼ teaspoon sea salt
- ⅛ teaspoons black pepper

Vegetable Stir-Fry:
- 1 lime, juiced
- 1 head red cabbage, shredded
- 1 cup shredded carrots
- 2 red bell peppers, cut into very thin strips
- Spice blend (remaining amount)
- Dash of hot sauce (optional)
- 4 mandarin oranges, segmented
- 2 tablespoons chopped fresh cilantro,

Prep

1. Combine all the ingredients for the spice blend and set aside.

Cook

2. Heat 1 tablespoon olive oil in a large skillet or wok over medium heat. Add 1 tablespoon of the spice blend and stir until fragrant, about 30 seconds. Add the ground turkey; cook and stir until browned on both sides and no pink remains. Remove the meat from the skillet.

3. To cook the vegetables, add the juice of 1 lime to the same skillet over medium heat. Using a wooden spoon, scrape the bottom of the pan to remove the cooked-on meat. Add the red cabbage, carrots, red bell pepper strips, and the remaining spice blend. Cook for 3 to 5 minutes, stirring occasionally. Add the hot sauce to the vegetables if desired, and mix well.

Serve

4. Plate the stir-fry mixture and top with turkey; garnish with fresh cilantro and mandarin segments.

Turkey Tahini
Bowl

Ingredients

Vegetables:

- 4 cups shredded red cabbage
- 4 cups arugula
- 1 cup diced red bell peppers
- 1 lime, juiced
- ¼ cup fresh cilantro, chopped
- ¼ teaspoon sea salt
- ⅛ teaspoon black pepper

Tahini Sauce:

- ¼ cup tahini
- 3 tablespoons lemon juice
- ⅛ teaspoon sea salt

Turkey:

- 1 tablespoon olive oil
- 1½ tablespoons dried cilantro
- 1½ teaspoons ground cumin
- 1½ teaspoons ground garlic
- 2 pounds ground turkey
- Fresh cilantro (for garnish)

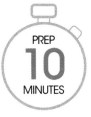

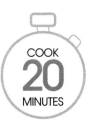

Prep

1. Combine the red cabbage, arugula, and red bell peppers. Add the juice of 1 lime with the cilantro, sea salt, and black pepper; toss to combine thoroughly.

2. In a small bowl, combine the tahini, lemon juice, and sea salt; mix well and set aside.

Cook

3. Heat 1 tablespoon olive oil in a large skillet or wok over medium heat. Add the dried cilantro, cumin, and garlic; stir until fragrant, about 30 seconds. Add the ground turkey; cook and stir until browned and no pink remains.

Serve

4. Plate the fresh vegetable mixture and top with turkey; garnish with tahini sauce and fresh cilantro.

⋽M Success Stories

Lindsay B., Wenonah, NJ

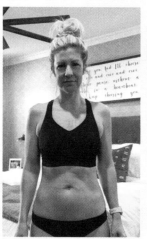 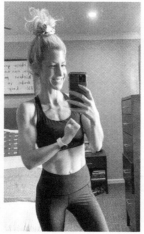

Rounds	Age	Weight Loss
5	40	15

When I joined E2M fitness, I was a full-time working mom with two kids. The daily grind was exhausting. At the end of the day, my "me time" was sitting on the couch with multiple glasses of wine, snacks, and binging shows till the early morning hours. The program shifted my entire perspective on life. I learned how to work out first thing, eat healthy (in a culture that makes it very confusing), and be more disciplined while giving myself grace because perfection doesn't exist.

What does the E2M community mean to you?
The E2M community is the magic to this program.

Nassim E., Clarksville, MD

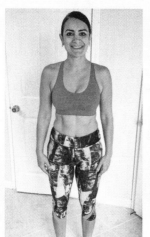 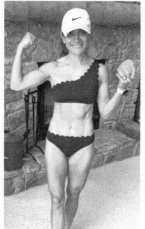

Rounds	Age	Weight Loss
10	44	15

I'm a super busy wife and mother of two that spends most of my time and energy serving others. When I started the program, I was working sixty-hour weeks and struggled to find time for myself. Once I started E2M fitness, I found that I'm happier and more successful in ALL aspects of my life. I've found the confidence to shift my professional path to explore my passions.

What is your biggest E2M fitness accomplishment?
My consistency. I've worked out at least thirty minutes a day for over two years!

Asian Turkey Bok Choy
and Mushrooms

Ingredients

Turkey:
- 2 pounds turkey breast, diced
- 2 tablespoons olive oil, divided
- 2 tablespoons Asian Spice Blend (see page 111)

Vegetables:
- 1 lime, zested and juiced
- 1½ pounds bok choy, chopped
- 1 cup sliced mushrooms
- 1 red chili pepper, seeded and chopped
- 2 tablespoons Asian Spice Blend (see page 111)
- 1 cup peanuts, chopped
- 4 lime wedges (for garnish)

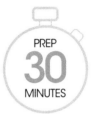

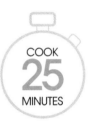

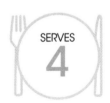

Prep

1. Combine all the ingredients for the Asian Spice Blend; mix well and set aside.

2. Put the turkey in a medium bowl; drizzle with 1 tablespoon of the olive oil, then toss to coat well. Add 2 tablespoons of the Asian Spice Blend, and mix well. Refrigerate for 30 minutes.

Cook

3. Pour the remaining 1 tablespoon of olive oil in a large pan over medium heat. Once the pan is hot, add the seasoned diced turkey breast. Continue cooking until the turkey is fully cooked and no pink remains. Remove from the pan and set aside. Cook in batches if the pan is not big enough.

4. In the same pan, squeeze the juice of 1 lime; scrape the pan with a wooden spoon to remove any cooked-on turkey. Add the bok choy, mushrooms, red chili pepper, lime zest, and the remaining 2 tablespoons of the Asian Spice Blend. Cook for 3 minutes, or until the vegetables are tender.

Serve

5. Divide the vegetable mixture between bowls; top with diced turkey. Garnish each serving with chopped peanuts and 1 lime wedge.

E2M Success Stories

Daisy R., Cherry Hill, NJ

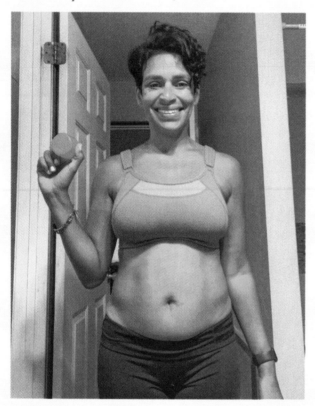
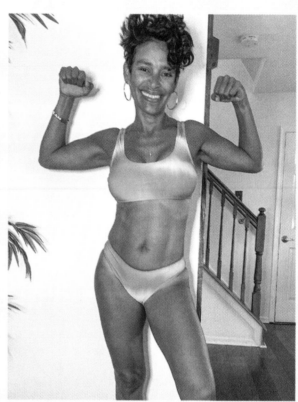

Rounds	Age	Weight Loss
1	52	20

Two years ago, I picked up bad habits out of boredom while working remotely. I started eating processed foods and drinking a few glasses of wine after work. The weight started creeping on, and I felt unmotivated to exercise. E2M fitness gave me the refocus needed and now I'm twenty pounds lighter, with glowing skin, sleeping through the night, and full of energy.

What were you hoping to gain from your E2M fitness experience?
I was hesitant to sign up because it was an online platform, and I had already tried something similar. I decided to trust my friend who was excited about her results. Now I have an E2M fit family, coaches, and tools to support me with my new lifestyle.

What is your favorite type of workout?
My favorite workouts are the E2M circuits. They are short but effective.

Garlic Ginger Turkey
Stir-Fry

Ingredients

Turkey:
- 2 pounds turkey breast cutlets, diced
- 1 tablespoon olive oil
- 2 tablespoons stir-fry sauce (recipe below)

Vegetables:
- 1 lime, juiced
- 4 cups shredded cabbage
- 1 cup carrots, shredded
- 1 cup thinly sliced red bell pepper
- Stir-fry sauce (remaining amount)
- 1 cup cashews, chopped
- ¼ cup fresh parsley, chopped

Stir-Fry Sauce:
- 2 tablespoons olive oil
- 3 tablespoons rice vinegar
- 1 teaspoon ground garlic
- ½ teaspoon ground ginger
- 1 tablespoon sesame seeds
- 1 lime, zested and juiced

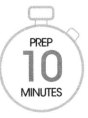

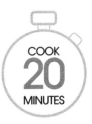

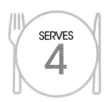

Prep

1. Prepare the stir-fry sauce by combining all ingredients together; mix thoroughly, then set aside.

2. Toss the diced turkey in 2 tablespoons of the stir-fry sauce.

Cook

3. Heat 1 tablespoon olive oil in a large skillet or wok over medium heat. Add the diced turkey; cook and stir until browned and fully cooked, approximately 5 to 8 minutes on each side. Remove the meat from the skillet.

4. To cook the vegetables, squeeze the juice of 1 lime into the same skillet over medium heat. Using a wooden spoon, scrape the bottom of the pan to remove the cooked-on bits of meat. Add the cabbage, carrots, red bell pepper, and the remaining stir-fry sauce. Cook for 3 to 5 minutes, stirring occasionally.

Serve

5. Plate the stir-fry vegetables, and top with diced turkey breast; garnish with chopped cashews and fresh parsley.

Turkey Meatloaf
Muffins

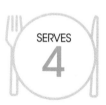

PREP
20
MINUTES

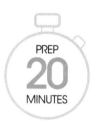

COOK
50
MINUTES

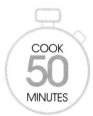

SERVES
4

Ingredients

Meatloaf Muffins:
- 2 pounds ground turkey
- ½ cup diced onion
- 1½ teaspoons ground garlic
- 1½ teaspoons smoked paprika
- 1 teaspoon ground mustard
- ¼ teaspoon sea salt
- ⅛ teaspoon black pepper
- Cooking oil spray
- 4 cups spring mix

Spicy Roasted Pepper Sauce:
- 6 red bell peppers
- ½ jalapeño
- ½ cup water
- 2 teaspoons Italian seasoning
- 2 teaspoons sea salt
- 1 teaspoon black pepper

Cauliflower Puree:
- 4 cups cooked cauliflower rice
- 1½ teaspoons olive oil
- ¼ teaspoon sea salt
- ⅛ teaspoon black pepper

Prep

1. Preheat the oven to 350 degrees. Line a baking sheet with parchment paper or spray with cooking oil.

2. Cut the red bell peppers and jalapeño in half; remove the seeds and stems. Put the prepared red bell peppers and jalapeño on the baking sheet to roast.

Cook

3. Roast the peppers for 20 minutes. Prepare the meatloaf while the peppers are baking.

4. Make the meatloaf in a large bowl by combining the ground turkey, onion, garlic, smoked paprika, mustard, sea salt, and black pepper; mix thoroughly. Generously spray each well of a muffin tin with cooking oil. Divide the meat mixture into a 6-well muffin tin. Bake the meatloaf muffins for 30 minutes.

5. When the peppers are finished baking, allow them to cool slightly, then put them in a blender or food processor; add the water, Italian seasoning, sea salt, and black pepper. Blend until smooth to make red pepper sauce and set aside.

6. Combine the cooked cauliflower with the olive oil, sea salt, and black pepper; blend with an immersion blender or food processor until smooth. Put the pureed cauliflower in a ziplock bag, and cut off the corner to make a piping bag.

7. After the muffins have baked for 30 minutes, remove from the oven and allow to cool. Top with the cauliflower puree and red pepper sauce. Return the muffin pan to the oven; continue to cook 5 minutes more, or until the internal temperature reaches 165 degrees. Remove from the oven; let cool before removing from the tin.

Serve

8. Plate spring mix and top with the meatloaf muffins. These also pair well with zucchini zoodles.

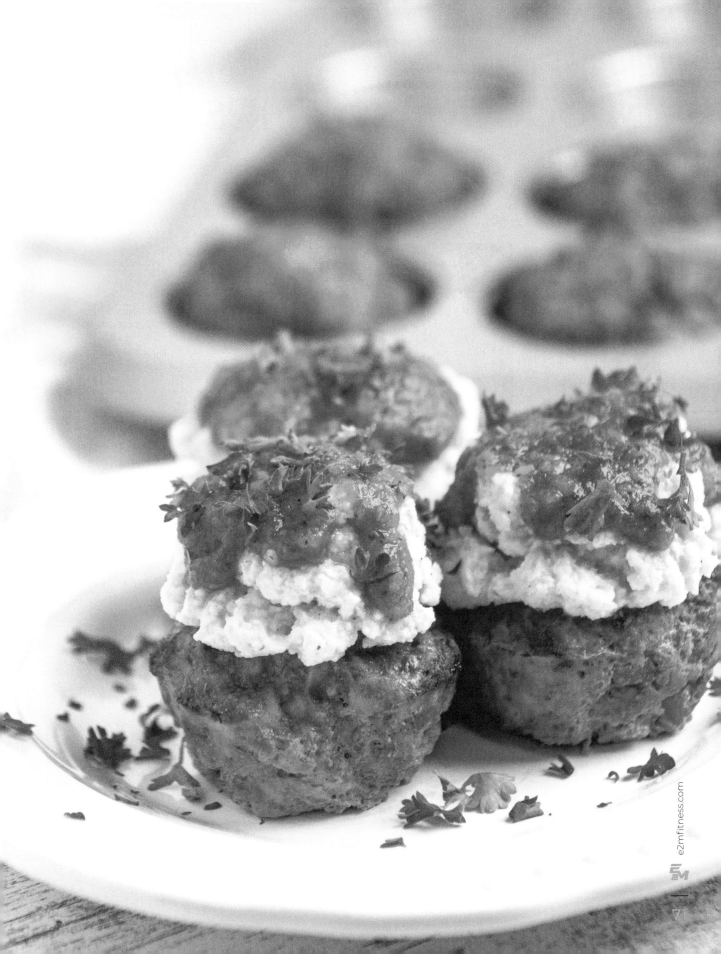

≡M Success Stories

Cliff H., Taylors, SC

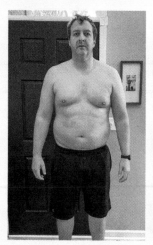 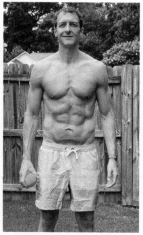

Rounds	Age	Weight Loss
3	42	85

My biggest accomplishments through E2M fitness have been losing eighty-five pounds, getting off blood pressure meds, going from around 30 percent body fat to 10.3 percent. I initially wanted to lose weight, but I've received so much more than just weight loss because of this program.

What is your favorite type of workout?
I love all the EC workouts: Sunday Thunder, Murder Monday, Tuesday and Saturday Burns, and Wednesday Sizzle.

What does the E2M community mean to you?
It's a great space to interact with awesome people who have similar goals!

Savanah D., Charleston, SC

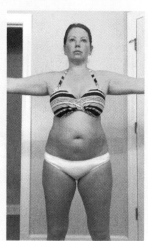 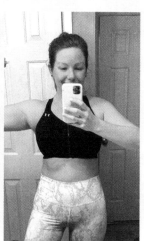

Rounds	Age	Weight Loss
2	36	16

I quit smoking in March 2021 for an elective surgery and gained about twenty pounds when my metabolism quit on me. In May 2021, I found E2M fitness and have enjoyed every minute of it since. I just completed my anniversary round.

What did you want to change about your lifestyle?
I was eating and drinking like a king all day, every day. I needed some control, portion size, and fasting in my life.

Non-Scale Victory (NSV)!
My mental health, the friendships, the clear skin.

Chicken

Cajun Chicken
and Broccoli Rice

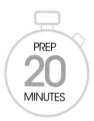

PREP
20
MINUTES

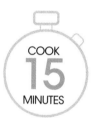

COOK
15
MINUTES

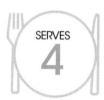

SERVES
4

Ingredients

Cajun Chicken:

- 2 pounds chicken breast
- 1 tablespoon olive oil
- Cooking oil spray

- 1½ tablespoons Cajun Blend (see page 109)

Broccoli Rice:

- 8 cups broccoli florets or 2 heads broccoli
- 1 teaspoon kosher salt

- 1 cup diced red pepper
- 1 teaspoon black pepper
- 1 teaspoon ground garlic

Prep

1. For the Cajun Blend, combine all the ingredients and mix well; store in an airtight container.

2. If using larger chicken breasts, butterfly the meat before cutting the chicken breasts lengthwise into thinner cutlets; put them in a large bowl with the olive oil. Sprinkle 1½ tablespoons of the Cajun Blend on the chicken; toss to coat evenly.

3. To prepare the riced broccoli, use a sharp knife to cut the broccoli into 1-inch florets. Put the florets in a food processor (work in batches if needed); pulse until the broccoli resembles the size of rice, scraping the sides of the bowl as necessary. Set aside.

Cook

4. Heat a large pan over medium heat; spray with cooking oil. Cook the chicken for 5 minutes, or until the edges turn white; flip and cook for another 4 to 5 minutes, until the chicken reaches an internal temperature of 165 degrees. Transfer to a plate, cover with foil, and let rest for 5 minutes.

5. Use the same pan over medium heat, and spray again with cooking oil. Add the broccoli rice and red pepper in one layer; cook until it becomes bright green and tender, 2 to 3 minutes. Season with the kosher salt, garlic, and black pepper.

Serve

6. Put the broccoli rice on the bottom of each bowl, and top with the Cajun chicken.

Lemon Basil
Stuffed Chicken

Ingredients

Avocado Salsa:
- 2 avocados, peeled and diced
- 1 lemon, zested and juiced
- 1 tablespoon chopped fresh basil
- ½ teaspoon sea salt
- ¼ teaspoon black pepper

Chicken and Vegetables:
- 4 cups spinach
- 1 bunch fresh asparagus, trimmed
- 2 pounds chicken breast or tenders
- Small skewers or toothpicks
- Cooking oil spray
- Lemon Basil Seasoning (see page 109)
- 4 cups spring mix (serving option)

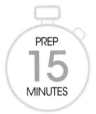

PREP
15
MINUTES

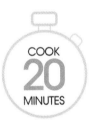

COOK
20
MINUTES

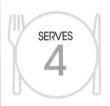

SERVES
4

Prep

1. For the Lemon Basil Seasoning, combine all the ingredients and mix well.

2. Prepare the avocado salsa in a bowl by combining the avocado, lemon zest, lemon juice, basil, sea salt, and black pepper; mix together. Cover with plastic wrap and refrigerate.

3. Chop up the spinach and asparagus into bite-size pieces; set aside.

4. Preheat the oven to 400 degrees. Line a sheet pan with parchment paper or spray with cooking oil.

5. Cut a pocket into the chicken along the side of the breast or tender. If using larger chicken breasts, butterfly the meat for quicker cooking. Stuff the asparagus and spinach into the opening in the chicken. Use a small skewer to hold closed. If extra stuffing is left over, sauté it in a pan over medium heat and serve as a side.

6. Spray the chicken with cooking oil; sprinkle both sides with Lemon Basil Seasoning to fully coat the chicken. Put the chicken on the prepared pan.

Cook

7. Bake for 20 to 25 minutes, or until chicken reaches an internal temperature of 165 degrees.

Serve

8. Serve the stuffed chicken over spring mix. Top with the avocado salsa.

Meal prep idea:

Prepare the chicken, let cool, and divide into airtight containers. Store in the refrigerator for up to three days.

e2mfitness.com

Chicken Chia Meatballs
with Roasted Red Pepper Sauce

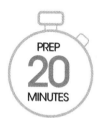

PREP
20
MINUTES

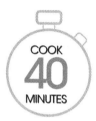

COOK
40
MINUTES

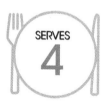

SERVES
4

Ingredients

Chicken Chia Meatballs:
- 2 pounds ground chicken
- 2 teaspoons ground garlic
- 2 teaspoons Italian seasoning
- 1 tablespoon sea salt
- 2 teaspoons black pepper
- ¼ cup chia seeds
- 1 tablespoon avocado oil

Roasted Red Pepper Sauce:
- 6 red bell peppers
- ½ jalapeño
- ½ cup water
- 2 teaspoons Italian seasoning
- 2 teaspoons sea salt
- 1 teaspoon black pepper

Noodles:
- Cooking oil spray
- 6 medium zucchini, spiralized, or buy premade zoodles
- ⅛ teaspoon sea salt
- ⅛ teaspoon black pepper

Prep

1. Prepare the meatballs in a large bowl by combining the ground chicken, garlic, Italian seasoning, sea salt, black pepper, and chia seeds; mix thoroughly. Refrigerate for 10 minutes so the chia can absorb the moisture; the seeds will act like glue to bind the meatballs. Preheat the oven to 350 degrees. Line a baking sheet with parchment paper.

2. For each meatball, scoop a rounded tablespoon of the meat mixture, about 1 ounce, and shape into a ball; put the meatballs on a plate.

3. To prepare the roasted red pepper sauce, cut the red bell peppers and jalapeño in half; remove the seeds and stems. Put the prepared red bell peppers and jalapeño on the baking sheet.

Cook

4. Bake the red peppers and jalepeno peppers for 20 minutes. When they are finished, allow the roasted peppers to cool slightly and put them in a blender or food processor with the water, Italian seasoning, sea salt, and black pepper; blend until smooth.

5. Heat the avocado oil in a large skillet over medium heat. Add the meatballs to the hot pan; brown on both sides, then add the roasted red pepper sauce to the pan. Continue cooking on medium heat for 8 to 12 minutes, until the meatballs reach an internal temperature of 165 degrees.

6. Heat a separate pan over high heat; spray with cooking oil. Sauté the zucchini noodles for 2 minutes; season with the sea salt and black pepper.

Serve

7. Plate the zucchini noodles; add the chicken meatballs and sauce.

Meal prep idea:
Prepare the meatballs, let cool, and divide into airtight containers. Store in the refrigerator for up to three days. You can also freeze the meatballs in an airtight freezer-safe container.

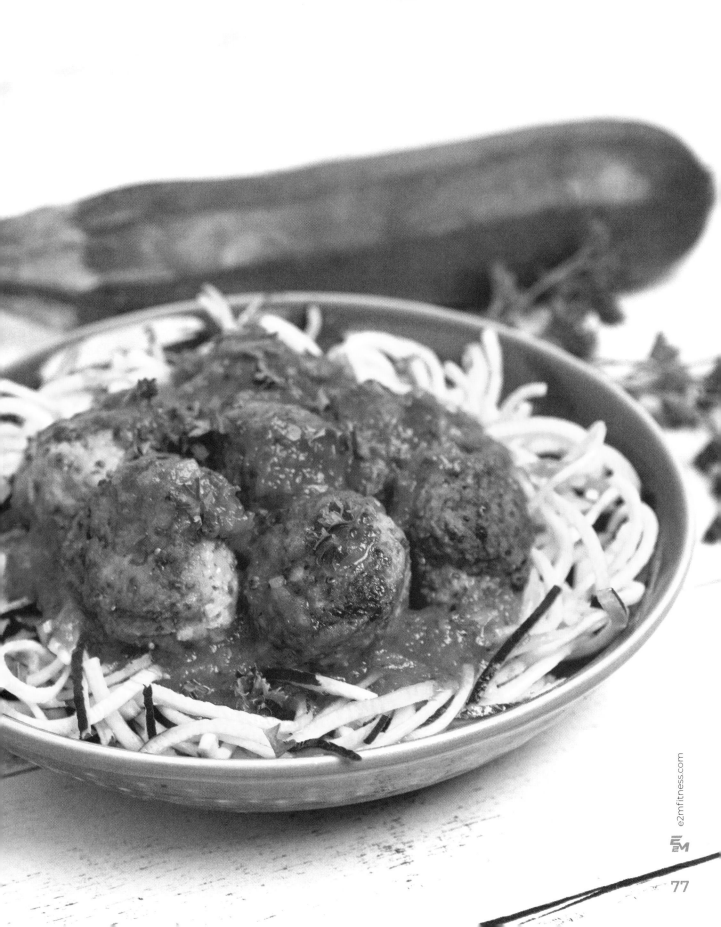

Evans J., Jupiter, FL

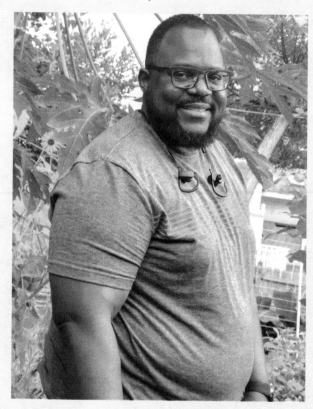 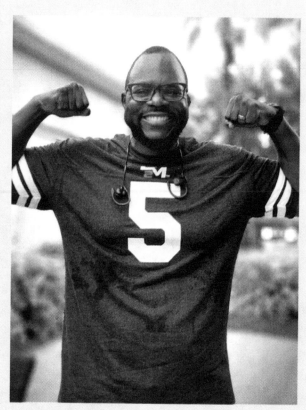

Rounds	Age	Weight Loss
5	43	80

The E2M program provided the tools needed in order to gain more confidence in myself, changed my eating habits, and made my workouts more effective.

What were you hoping to gain from your E2M experience?
I'm hoping to motivate more people to take charge of their health. E2M fitness is not a diet program, it's a lifestyle change. I am a result of trusting the process.

Non-Scale Victory (NSV)!
I'm no longer prediabetic.

Spicy BBQ Chicken
with "Ranch" Vegetables

Ingredients

Chicken:
- 2 pounds diced chicken breast
- 2 tablespoons Spicy BBQ Rub (recipe to the right)
- Cooking oil spray
- 1 tablespoon olive oil

Vegetables:
- 2 cups diced zucchini
- 2 cups sliced red bell peppers
- 2 cups sliced button mushrooms
- 1½ tablespoons olive oil
- 2 cups quartered broccoli florets
- 3 tablespoons "Ranch" Seasoning (see page 107)

Spicy BBQ Rub:
- 1 tablespoon smoked paprika
- 1 teaspoon chili powder
- 1 teaspoon ground garlic
- ¼ teaspoon ground cumin
- ¼ teaspoon ground mustard
- ¼ teaspoon sea salt
- ⅛ teaspoon black pepper
- ⅛ teaspoon ground cayenne pepper
- ⅛ teaspoon crushed red pepper
- ⅛ teaspoon chipotle seasoning

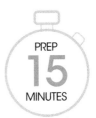

PREP
15
MINUTES

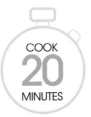

COOK
20
MINUTES

SERVES
4

Prep

1. Make the Spicy BBQ Rub in a small bowl by combining the listed ingredients; mix well. Repeat for the "Ranch" Seasoning in a second small bowl. Store any leftover blends in separate airtight containers.

2. Prepare the chicken in a large bowl by combining the diced chicken breast, 1 tablespoon olive oil, and 2 tablespoons Spicy BBQ Rub; mix well. Cover and marinate in the refrigerator for 30 minutes.

3. Preheat the oven to 425 degrees. Line a sheet pan with parchment paper.

4. To make the vegetables, combine the zucchini, red bell peppers, mushrooms, and broccoli in a large bowl with 1½ tablespoons olive oil and 3 tablespoons of the "Ranch" Seasoning. Toss to coat evenly; put the vegetables on the sheet pan.

Cook

5. Bake the vegetables for 6 to 8 minutes, or until the vegetables are tender.

6. While the vegetables are in the oven, heat a large nonstick skillet over medium heat; spray with cooking oil. Add the diced chicken and cook for 4 to 6 minutes, or until chicken reaches an internal temperature of 165 degrees.

Serve

7. Plate the chicken and serve with the roasted vegetables.

Meal prep idea:
Prepare the chicken and vegetables, let cool, and divide into airtight containers. Store in the refrigerator for up to three days.

e2mfitness.com

Lemon Chicken
with Green Bean Almondine

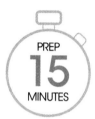

PREP
15
MINUTES

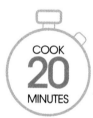

COOK
20
MINUTES

SERVES
4

Meal prep idea:
Prepare the chicken and green beans, let cool, and divide into airtight containers. Store in the refrigerator for up to three days.

Ingredients

Lemon Chicken:

- Cooking oil spray
- 2 tablespoons olive oil
- 2 teaspoons dried oregano
- 2 teaspoons ground garlic
- 2 teaspoons sea salt
- 1 teaspoon dried thyme
- ½ teaspoon black pepper
- 1 lemon, zested and juiced
- 2 pounds chicken tenderloins
- 1 lemon, cut into 6 slices (optional)

Green Bean Almondine:

- 2 tablespoons olive oil, divided
- ½ cup slivered almonds
- 2 pounds green beans
- 1 tablespoon ground garlic
- ¼ cup water
- 2 teaspoons sea salt

Prep

1. Heat the oven to 400 degrees. Prepare a baking dish by spraying with cooking oil.

2. Prepare the lemon chicken in a large bowl by first combining the olive oil, oregano, garlic, sea salt, thyme, black pepper, lemon zest, and lemon juice to create a thick marinade paste. Add the chicken tenderloins to the marinade; mix well to coat evenly.

Cook

3. Put the chicken in the prepared baking dish; if using the optional lemon slices, nestle those between the tenderloins. Bake for 10 minutes, then baste the chicken by spooning the pan juices over the meat; bake for another 10 minutes, or until the internal temperature of the chicken is 165 degrees.

4. In a large pan, toast the almonds by first heating 1 tablespoon olive oil over medium heat. Add the almonds and toast until golden brown, about 2 minutes; set aside.

5. Heat 1 tablespoon olive oil in the same pan over medium-high heat; add the green beans and garlic. Cook for 2 to 3 minutes; add ¼ cup water to the pan and cover. Cook for an additional 3 to 5 minutes, or until the beans are cooked. Stir in the toasted almonds and sea salt, continuing to stir for another minute to combine everything.

Serve

6. Plate the chicken with the sautéed greens beans.

Oven-Roasted Chicken
with Kale

Ingredients

Chicken:

- 2 pounds chicken breast or tenders
- ¼ cup whole grain or Dijon mustard
- 2 tablespoons Everything Seasoning (see page 111)
- Cooking oil spray

Kale:

- 8 cups chopped kale
- 2 cups chopped sweet peppers
- 1 tablespoon olive oil
- 1 teaspoon sea salt
- ½ teaspoon black pepper
- ½ teaspoon ground garlic
- 2 avocados, peeled and sliced

Prep

1. For the Everything Seasoning, combine all the ingredients and mix well; store in an airtight container.

2. In a bowl, coat the chicken with the mustard and 2 tablespoons of Everything Seasoning. Toss to combine. Refrigerate for at least 30 minutes to marinate and impart flavor.

3. Preheat the oven to 400 degrees. Line a sheet pan with parchment paper.

4. Prepare the kale in a large bowl by combining the kale and sweet peppers, then add the olive oil, sea salt, black pepper, and garlic; toss to coat evenly. Spread out on the sheet pan.

Cook

5. Heat a large nonstick pan over high heat. Thoroughly spray the pan with cooking oil; sear the marinated chicken for 1 minute per side, then transfer to the sheet pan with the kale and peppers. If using larger chicken breasts, butterfly the meat for quicker cooking.

6. Bake at 400 degrees for 10 to 15 minutes, or until the chicken reaches an internal temperature of 165 degrees and the kale and peppers are slightly brown.

Serve

7. Plate the chicken and roasted vegetables, then add the avocado slices.

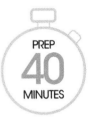

PREP
40
MINUTES

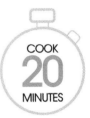

COOK
20
MINUTES

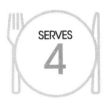

SERVES
4

Meal prep idea:

Prepare the chicken and vegetables, let cool, and divide into airtight containers. Store in the refrigerator for up to three days.

Mediterranean Chicken
with Roasted Vegetables

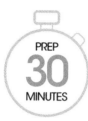

PREP
30
MINUTES

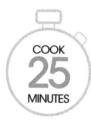

COOK
25
MINUTES

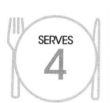

SERVES
4

Ingredients

Olive Tapenade:
- 1 cup diced black olives
- 1 tablespoon red wine vinegar
- 1 tablespoon olive oil
- ½ teaspoon Mediterranean Blend (see page 106)

Vegetables:
- 1 bunch asparagus, trimmed
- 2 zucchini
- 2 red bell peppers
- 1 tablespoon olive oil
- 1 tablespoon lemon juice
- 1 tablespoon Mediterranean Blend

Chicken:
- 2 pounds chicken breast or tenders
- Cooking oil spray
- 4 cups spring mix or lettuce blend
- Mediterranean Blend (remaining amount)

Prep

1. Combine all the ingredients for the Mediterranean Spice Blend; mix thoroughly.

2. Preheat the oven to 400 degrees. Line a sheet pan with parchment paper or spray with cooking oil.

3. For the olive tapenade, combine the olives, red wine vinegar, olive oil, and ½ teaspoon of the Mediterranean Spice Blend in a blender. Blend until well combined. Tapenade can be chunky in texture. Set aside.

4. Chop the asparagus, zucchini, and red bell peppers into large dice; combine in a bowl. Drizzle the olive oil over the vegetables, add the lemon juice, and toss to coat evenly. Sprinkle 1 tablespoon of the Mediterranean Spice Blend over the vegetables, and toss once more until the seasonings are evenly distributed.

5. Spray both sides of the chicken breast with cooking oil. Sprinkle the remaining Mediterranean Spice Blend on both sides of chicken to fully coat.

Cook

6. Put the chicken on the pan; if using a large breast, butterfly the meat for quicker cooking. Spread the vegetables around the chicken on the sheet pan, making sure not to overcrowd the pan. Roast at 400 degrees for 20 to 25 minutes, or until the chicken reaches an internal temperature of 165 degrees.

Serve

7. Plate the spring mix; top with the chicken and roasted vegetables, then the olive tapenade.

Meal prep idea:
Prepare the chicken and vegetables, let cool, and divide into airtight containers. Store in the refrigerator for up to three days.

e2mfitness.com

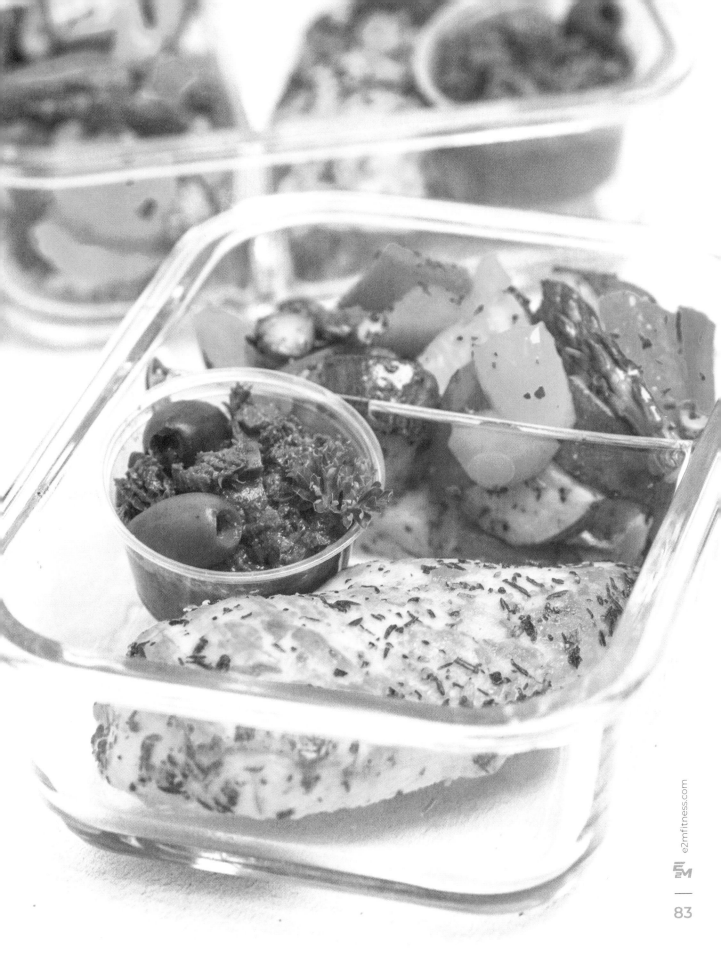

Success Stories

Karen M., Goose Creek, SC

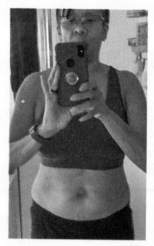
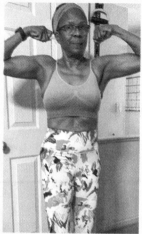

Rounds	Age	Weight Loss
2	66	20

I started the E2M program at sixty-five years young with joint issues, stiffness, and needing to lose weight. As an ICU nurse, I sought results, and I knew the program worked from witnessing my son come off insulin in one round. The community is amazing and so supportive all the time, which is rare.

What is your biggest E2M fitness accomplishment?
I've changed physically and socially. As an introvert, I've formed lasting relationships within this E2M community.

Non-Scale Victory (NSV)!
I went from wearing a size 8 to wearing a size 4.

Sibylle T., Okemos, MI

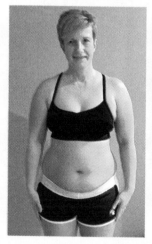
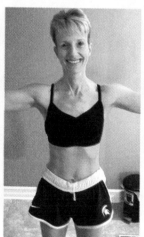

Rounds	Age	Weight Loss
4	46	69

I'm the healthiest, fittest, and happiest I've ever been in all my life. I didn't know what to expect. Initially, I aimed for weight loss but once I joined, I realized this will be my lifestyle.

What did you want to change about your lifestyle?
Increase my energy and feeling good.

Non-Scale Victory (NSV)!
I'm out of the obese range with my BMI, off reflux and antidepressant meds, body fat range at an athletic level, and I can finally sleep at night.

Chicken Lettuce Tacos
with Pineapple Slaw

Ingredients

Pineapple Slaw:
- 1 cup diced pineapple, fresh or canned (drained)
- 1 lime, zested and juiced
- 1 teaspoon olive oil
- 1 teaspoon rice vinegar
- ¼ teaspoon sea salt
- ¼ teaspoon black pepper
- 2 (8-ounce) packages prepared broccoli slaw or cabbage slaw

Guac Spread:
- 2 avocados
- 1 lime, zested and juiced
- ½ teaspoon chopped fresh cilantro
- ¼ teaspoon sea salt
- ¼ teaspoon ground cumin

Tacos:
- 1 tablespoon olive oil
- Taco Seasoning (recipe below)
- 2 pounds chicken breast or tenders
- Hot sauce, green or red (optional)
- 1 head bib lettuce
- 1 lime, zested and juiced
- Fresh cilantro (for garnish)

Taco Seasoning:
- 1 tablespoon chili powder
- 1 teaspoon ground cumin
- 1 teaspoon sea salt
- ½ teaspoon ground cayenne pepper
- ½ teaspoon ground garlic

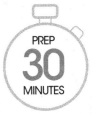

PREP
30
MINUTES

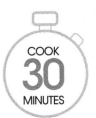

COOK
30
MINUTES

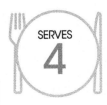

SERVES
4

Prep

1. Prepare the pineapple slaw by combining the pineapple in a bowl with the zest and juice of one lime and the olive oil, rice vinegar, sea salt, and black pepper; mix to combine. Add the broccoli slaw and toss to coat evenly. Marinate in the refrigerator for at least 30 minutes.

2. To make the guac spread, cut the avocados in half, remove the seed, spoon out avocado flesh into a bowl, and mash with a fork. Add the zest and juice of one lime, fresh cilantro, sea salt, and cumin. Set aside and cover with an airtight lid to prevent browning.

3. For the Taco Seasoning, whisk together all the ingredients in a small bowl. Set aside.

Cook

4. Pour 1 tablespoon olive oil into a dutch oven or deep pot over medium heat, and spread to coat the bottom. Add all of the Taco Seasoning; heat until you start to smell the spices, being careful not to burn them. Add the chicken to the pot; stir to coat in spices.

5. Pour in enough water to completely cover the chicken; bring to a boil. Continue boiling for 20 minutes, or until the chicken reaches an internal temperature of 165 degrees. Remove the chicken from the broth; allow to cool.

6. Shred the chicken with two forks by pulling apart, or use a hand mixer to shred. Add hot sauce if desired and toss to combine.

Serve

7. Plate the lettuce leaves as the taco "shell"; layer the slaw, then shredded chicken. Top with guac spread, lime zest, lime juice, and chopped cilantro.

Meal prep idea:
Prepare the chicken, let cool, and divide into airtight containers. Keep in the refrigerator for up to three days.

e2mfitness.com

Ginger Garlic Chicken
Stir-Fry

PREP
30
MINUTES

COOK
20
MINUTES

SERVES
4

Ingredients

Stir-Fry Marinade:

- 1 tablespoon dried basil
- 1 tablespoon ground garlic
- 1½ teaspoons ground ginger
- 3 tablespoons olive oil
- 3 tablespoons rice vinegar
- 1 lime, zested and juiced
- 1 teaspoon crushed red pepper (optional)
- ½ teaspoon ground cayenne pepper (optional)

Chicken and Vegetables:

- 2 pounds chicken breast or tenders
- Cooking oil spray
- 1 tablespoon lemon juice
- 1 cup shredded carrots
- 1 red bell pepper, diced
- 2 cups shredded purple cabbage
- 1 tablespoon chopped fresh cilantro,
- 1 lime, zested and juiced
- ½ cup peanuts, chopped

Prep

1. Prepare the stir-fry marinade in a bowl by combining the basil, garlic, ginger, olive oil, rice vinegar, lime zest, and lime juice, including any optional crushed red pepper or cayenne, if desired.

2. Dice the chicken into bite-size pieces; add to the marinade and toss to coat evenly. Marinate in the refrigerator for at least 30 minutes before cooking.

Cook

3. Heat a large pan over medium heat; spray with cooking oil. Add the marinated chicken to the pan and sear on one side. Flip and continue to cook until the chicken reaches an internal temperature of 165 degrees. Remove the chicken from the pan.

4. Using the same pan over medium heat to cook the vegetables, pour in the lemon juice, and using a wooden spoon, scrape the bottom of the pan to remove any cooked-on food to create a sauce. Add the carrots, red bell pepper, and purple cabbage. Sauté on medium heat until the vegetables are tender.

Serve

5. Plate the stir-fry veggies, top with the chicken, then garnish with fresh cilantro, lime zest, lime juice, and chopped peanuts.

Meal prep idea:
Prepare the chicken, let cool, and divide into airtight containers. Store stir-fry vegetables in a separate gallon plastic bag or airtight container. Keep in the refrigerator for up to three days.

e2mfitness.com

Chicken Satay
with Lemon Garlic Green Beans

Ingredients

Chicken:
- 10 wooden skewers
- 1½ pounds chicken breast or tenders
- 2 tablespoons chopped fresh parsley

Satay Marinade:
- 2 tablespoons olive oil
- 2 garlic cloves, minced
- ½ small red onion, small dice
- 2 teaspoons ground turmeric
- 1 teaspoon ground coriander
- 1 teaspoon chili powder
- 1½ teaspoons sea salt
- 1 teaspoon black pepper

Green Beans:
- Cooking oil spray
- 8 cups green beans, fresh or canned
- 1 lemon, zested and juiced
- 1 teaspoon ground garlic
- ¼ teaspoon sea salt
- ⅛ teaspoon black pepper

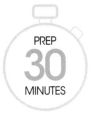

PREP
30
MINUTES

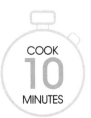

COOK
10
MINUTES

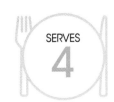

SERVES
4

Prep

1. Soak the skewers in water for 30 minutes prior to using to prevent splintering and burning.

2. Cut the chicken breast into strips about ½-inch wide and put in a bowl. Or if using chicken strips, remove the tendon and put in a bowl.

3. Prepare the marinade in a food processor by blending together the olive oil, garlic, red onion, turmeric, coriander, chili powder, sea salt, and black pepper. Add water if needed to thin out. Add the marinade to the chicken; toss to coat thoroughly. Refrigerate overnight or at least 4 hours.

Cook

4. Thread 1 strip of marinated chicken onto a bamboo skewer; repeat until finished.

5. Using an indoor grill pan or outdoor grill, heat to high heat and place the Chicken Satay skewers on an oiled grate for 3 to 4 minutes on each side, until the meat is fully cooked and the internal temperature is 165 degrees. While the chicken skewers are on the grill, start to cook the green beans.

6. To cook the green beans, heat a large skillet over medium-high heat; spray with cooking oil. Add the green beans, lemon zest, lemon juice, garlic, sea salt, and black pepper; sauté for 4 to 5 minutes.

Serve

7. Plate the skewers with the green beans; garnish with fresh parsley. These skewers pair well with the Thai Peanut Dressing for a delicious dipping sauce.

Spinach Artichoke
Stuffed Chicken

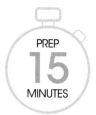

PREP
15
MINUTES

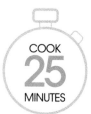

COOK
25
MINUTES

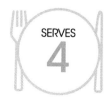

SERVES
4

Ingredients

Avocado Salsa:

- 2 avocados, peeled and diced
- 1 tablespoon chopped fresh cilantro
- 1 lemon, zested and juiced
- ½ teaspoon sea salt
- ¼ teaspoon black pepper

Chicken and Vegetables:

- 3 cups spinach
- 1 (14-ounce) can artichoke hearts, drained
- 1 teaspoon dried oregano, divided
- 1 teaspoon dried thyme, divided
- 1 lemon, zested and juiced
- 2 pounds chicken breast
- Small skewers or toothpicks
- Cooking oil spray
- 4 cups cauliflower rice, fresh or frozen

Prep

1. Prepare the avocado salsa in a bowl by combining the avocado, lemon zest, lemon juice, cilantro, sea salt, and black pepper; mix together. Cover with plastic wrap and refrigerate.

2. Preheat the oven to 400 degrees. Line a sheet pan with parchment paper or spray with cooking oil.

3. Chop the spinach and artichoke hearts into bite-size pieces. Add ½ teaspoon oregano, ½ teaspoon thyme, lemon zest, and lemon juice; toss to combine.

4. Cut a pocket into the chicken along the side of the breast. Spoon the artichoke and spinach mixture into the opening in the chicken. Use a small skewer or toothpick to hold closed.

Cook

5. Spray the chicken with cooking oil; sprinkle both sides with ½ teaspoon oregano and ½ teaspoon thyme to fully coat the chicken. Put the chicken on the prepared pan. Bake for 20 to 25 minutes or until the chicken reaches an internal temperature of 165 degrees.

6. Combine any remaining artichoke and spinach mixture with the cauliflower rice. Heat a pan to medium heat; spray with cooking oil. Sauté the cauliflower rice mixture for 5 to 8 minutes, until tender.

Serve

7. Plate the cauliflower rice; top with stuffed chicken and avocado salsa.

Chili-Lime Chicken
Burrito Bowl

Ingredients

Chicken:

- 1 tablespoon olive oil
- 1½ tablespoons Chili-Lime Seasoning (see page 106)
- 2 pounds diced chicken breast

- 2 avocados, peeled and sliced
- 2 tablespoons chopped fresh cilantro
- 1 lime, zested and juiced

Vegetables:

- 1 tablespoon olive oil
- Chili-Lime Seasoning (remaining amount)

- 1 red onion, diced
- 1 red bell pepper, diced
- 1 green bell pepper, diced

Prep

1. For the Chili-Lime Seasoning, combine all the ingredients and mix well.

Cook

2. Pour 1 tablespoon of the olive oil into a dutch oven or deep pot over medium heat. Add 1½ tablespoons of the Chili-Lime Seasoning; heat until you start to smell the spices, being careful not to burn them. Add the chicken, and stir to coat evenly in spices.

3. Pour in enough water to completely cover the chicken; bring to a boil. Continue boiling for 20 minutes, or until internal temperature reaches 165 degrees. Remove the chicken from the broth; allow to cool.

4. Shred the chicken with two forks by pulling apart, or use a hand mixer to shred. Tip: If using a hand mixer, use a kitchen towel to cover the bowl to prevent the chicken from coming out of the bowl. Add more spice blend, if desired.

5. While the chicken is boiling, heat a separate large pan over medium heat; add 1 tablespoon of olive oil and the remaining Chili-Lime Seasoning. Add the diced onion and bell peppers to the pan. Sauté until the vegetables are tender, 2 to 3 minutes.

Serve

6. Plate the shredded chicken and vegetables; top with diced avocado, fresh cilantro, and lime juice.

Chef tip:

Shredded chicken is a quick and easy way to prepare protein, especially for meal prep. You can mix and match spice blends to change up the flavor profile.

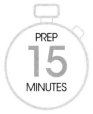

PREP
15
MINUTES

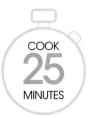

COOK
25
MINUTES

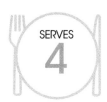

SERVES
4

Meal prep idea:

Prepare the chicken, let cool, and divide into airtight containers. Store vegetables in a separate plastic bag or airtight container. Keep in the refrigerator for up to three days.

Slow cooker option:

Pour 1 tablespoon oil and ½ to 1 cup water into slow cooker with chicken and dry seasonings. Cook on low for 6 hours.

e2mfitness.com

Success Stories

Eddie R., Hampton, VA

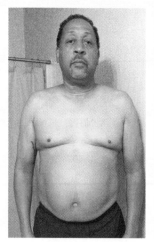
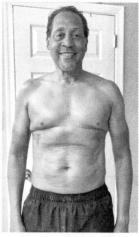

Rounds	Age	Weight Loss
10	55	45

I'm a prostate cancer warrior and survivor. Even with my complex medical issues, this program has helped me completely change my overall health profile.

What is your favorite type of workout?
My favorite types of workouts are the short, intense, extra credit burns offered by the coaches.

What is your biggest E2M fitness accomplishment?
My biggest accomplishments were my physical and mental transformation (ran 5 and 10Ks). After seeing my success, I influenced over seventy-five of my friends and family members to join the program.

Lauren A., St. Louis, MO

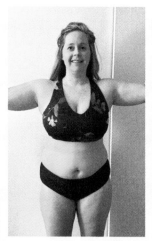
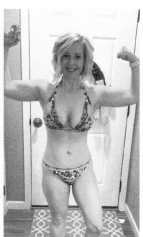

Rounds	Age	Weight Loss
8	34	40

It has not been easy. It still isn't easy, but let me tell you something: it's WORTH it! I cursed my way through every circuit, workout, and meal, yet I never gave up. As I look at the before pictures, I don't even know who that person is anymore. I never realized how I looked or how terrible I felt. Exercise has been the best medicine for me when it comes to my anxiety, sadness, and depression.

Non-Scale Victory (NSV)!
I have my confidence back! I feel absolutely incredible on the inside and outside!

"Ranch" Chicken
Meatballs

Ingredients

Meatballs:

- 2 pounds ground chicken
- 2 tablespoons Smoked Chili Seasoning (see page 109)
- 1 teaspoon sea salt
- 2 teaspoons "Ranch" Seasoning (see page 107)
- ¼ cup chia seeds
- Cooking oil spray

Salad:

- 4 cups arugula
- 4 cups shredded carrots
- 1 cup chopped celery
- 1 tablespoon "Ranch" Seasoning
- 1 tablespoon olive oil
- 1½ teaspoon rice vinegar

Prep

1. Make the Smoked Chili Seasoning in a small bowl by combining the listed ingredients; mix well. Repeat for the "Ranch" Seasoning in a second small bowl. Store any leftover blend in separate airtight containers.

2. To prepare the meatballs, combine the ground chicken, 2 tablespoons Smoked Chili Seasoning, 2 teaspoons "Ranch" Seasoning, sea salt, and chia seeds in a large bowl; mix thoroughly. Refrigerate for 10 minutes so the chia can absorb the moisture; the seeds will act like glue to bind the meatballs. Preheat the oven to 350 degrees. Line a sheet pan with parchment paper or spray with cooking oil.

3. Prepare the salad in a large bowl by combining the arugula, carrots, celery, 1 tablespoon "Ranch" Seasoning, olive oil, and rice vinegar.

4. For each meatball, scoop a rounded tablespoon of the meat mixture, about 1 ounce, and shape into a ball; put the meatballs on a plate.

Cook

5. Heat a large pan over medium heat; spray with cooking oil. Add the meatballs to the hot pan; brown on both sides. Transfer to the sheet pan. Bake for 8 to 12 minutes, until the meatballs reach an internal temperature of 165 degrees.

Serve

6. Plate the prepared salad, and top with "Ranch" meatballs.

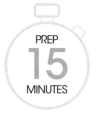

PREP
15
MINUTES

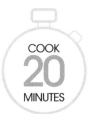

COOK
20
MINUTES

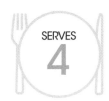

SERVES
4

Meal prep idea:
Prepare the chicken and vegetables, let cool, and divide into airtight containers. Store in the refrigerator for up to three days.

Note:
Chia seeds are a great vegan-friendly binder that can be used instead of eggs.

e2mfitness.com

Pineapple BBQ
Chicken

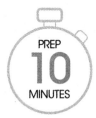

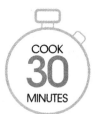

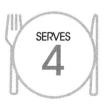

PREP **10** MINUTES

COOK **30** MINUTES

SERVES **4**

Ingredients

BBQ Sauce:
- 2 tablespoons apple cider vinegar
- 1 tablespoon red or green hot sauce
- 1 tablespoon olive oil
- ½ teaspoon smoked paprika
- 1 teaspoon chili powder

Vegetables:
- 8 cups shredded cabbage
- 1 cup diced pineapple
- 1 jalapeño, seeded and diced
- ½ cup diced red onion
- ¼ cup chopped fresh cilantro
- 2 limes, zested and juiced

Chicken:
- 1 tablespoon olive oil
- 2 teaspoons ground garlic
- 2 teaspoons smoked paprika
- 1½ teaspoons ground mustard
- 1½ teaspoons chili powder
- ¼ teaspoon sea salt
- ⅛ teaspoon black pepper
- 2 pounds chicken breast or tenders
- ⅛ teaspoon ground cayenne or crushed red pepper (optional)

Prep

1. Prepare the BBQ sauce by combining the apple cider vinegar, hot sauce, olive oil, paprika, and chili powder; set aside.

2. Combine the cabbage, pineapple, jalapeño, red onion, cilantro, lime zest, and lime juice; toss to combine.

Cook

3. Pour 1 tablespoon olive oil into a dutch oven or deep pot. Add the garlic, smoked paprika, mustard, chili powder, sea salt, and black pepper; heat until you start to smell the spices, being careful not to burn them. Add the chicken to the pot and coat it in spices.

4. Pour 3 to 4 cups of water into the pot, or enough to completely cover the chicken. Bring to a boil, then continue to boil for about 20 minutes, until the internal temperature of the chicken reaches 165 degrees. Remove the chicken from the broth; allow to cool.

5. Shred the chicken by pulling apart with two forks, or use a hand mixer to shred the meat. Toss the shredded chicken in the prepared BBQ sauce. Add optional cayenne or crushed red pepper for more heat.

Serve

6. Plate the cabbage mixture and top with the BBQ chicken.

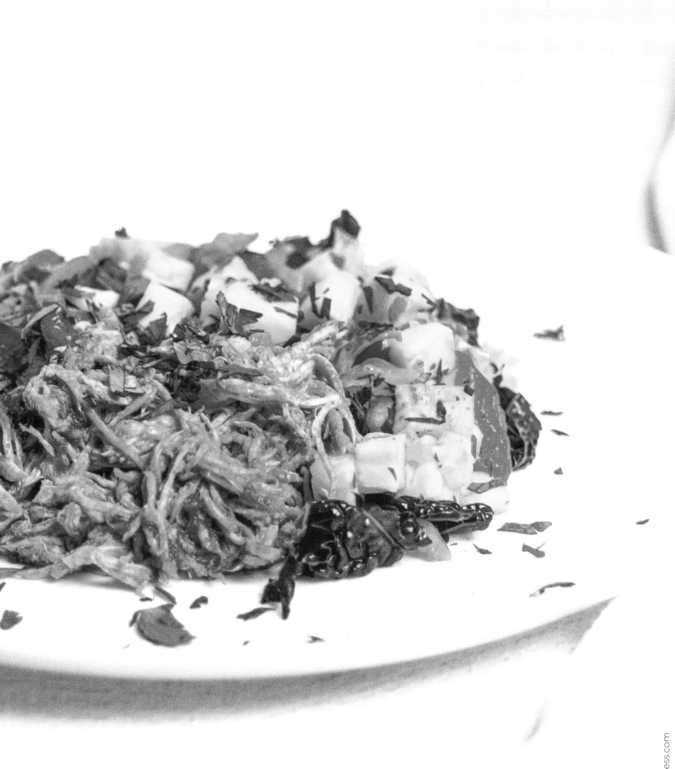

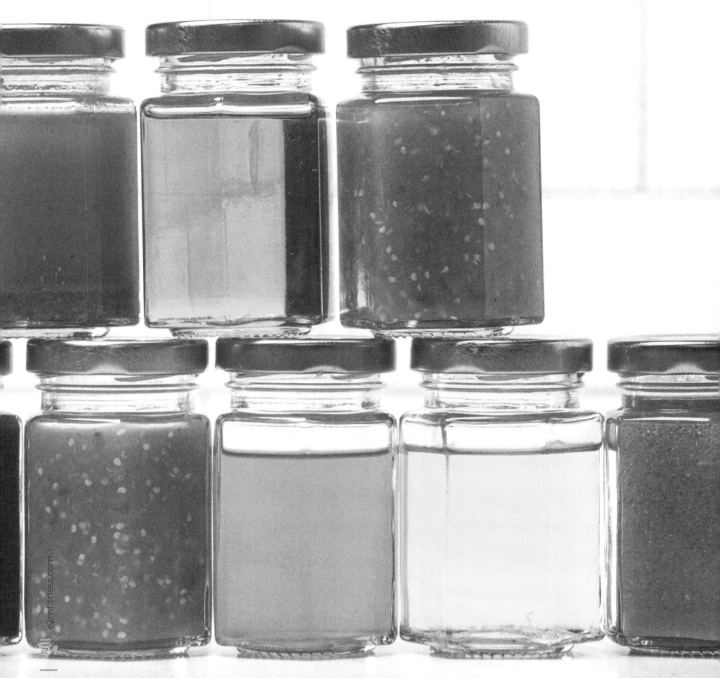

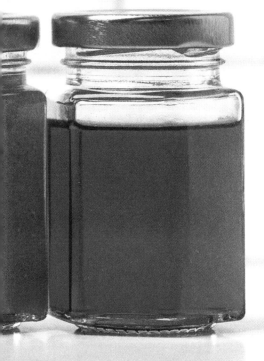

Dressings made from scratch are versatile and simple to make at home. Any of these dressing recipes can also be used as marinades for your proteins. These ingredients are used in many other recipes, so go ahead and buy in bulk to stock your pantry!

Another major benefit of homemade dressings is that they are free of preservatives, added sugars, and artificial flavorings. The more you know, the more you grow!

Dressings

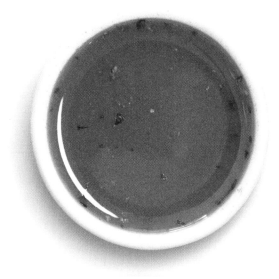

Italian Vinaigrette

½ cup extra-virgin olive oil
2 tablespoons red wine vinegar
1 teaspoon Dijon mustard
¼ teaspoon dried parsley
¼ teaspoon dried oregano
2 fresh garlic cloves, minced
⅛ teaspoon crushed red pepper
¼ teaspoon sea salt
⅛ teaspoon black pepper

Combine all ingredients in a mason jar, secure the lid, and shake. Store in an airtight container in the refrigerator for up to three days.

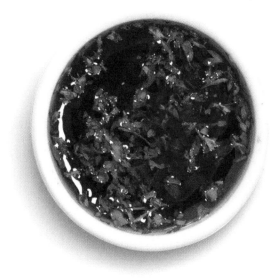

Chipotle Chimichurri Vinaigrette

½ cup extra-virgin olive oil
2 tablespoons fresh lime juice
2 tablespoons red wine vinegar
2 fresh garlic cloves, minced
¼ cup fresh flat leaf parsley, chopped
½ cup fresh cilantro, chopped
¼ teaspoon sea salt
¼ teaspoon ground chipotle seasoning

Combine all ingredients in a blender. Blend until smooth. Store in an airtight container in the refrigerator for up to three days.
Chef Note: pairs deliciously with chicken or beef.

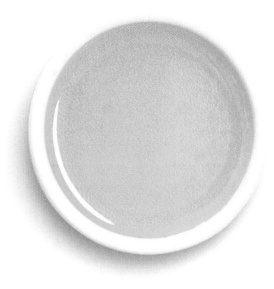

Lemon Vinaigrette

½ cup extra-virgin olive oil
3 tablespoons fresh lemon juice
1 teaspoon Dijon mustard
2 fresh garlic cloves, minced
¼ teaspoon sea salt
⅛ teaspoon black pepper

Combine all ingredients in a mason jar, secure the lid, and shake. Store in an airtight container in the refrigerator for up to three days.

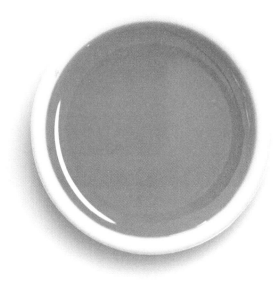

Red Pepper Dressing

½ cup extra-virgin olive oil
½ cup canned roasted red peppers, drained
¼ cup lemon juice
1 tablespoon Dijon mustard
1 fresh garlic clove, minced
½ teaspoon sea salt
¼ teaspoon black pepper

Combine all ingredients in a blender. Blend until smooth. Store in an airtight container in the refrigerator for up to three days.

Success Stories

Yari D., Summerville, SC

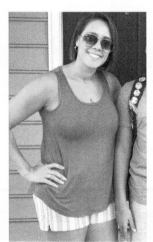
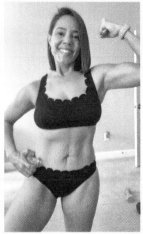

Rounds	Age	Weight Loss
14	37	21

The E2M program changed my life by teaching me that living a healthy lifestyle is what we all should want to attain. I worked out, but I didn't fuel my body accordingly. Through the program, I gained so much more than I could have ever imagined.

What is your favorite type of workout?
My favorite workouts are the circuit workouts, step aerobics/spinning for cardio, glutes, and upper body.

What is your biggest E2M fitness accomplishment?
Being able to motivate and inspire others to join me and watching them transform from the inside out!

Kevin E., Frewsburg, NY

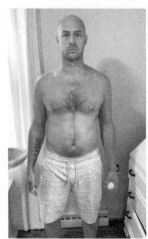
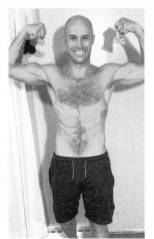

Rounds	Age	Weight Loss
1	35	20

E2M fitness has helped me set a positive example for my kids with a lifetime of healthy living surrounded by people who want to live the same way.

What did you want to change about your lifestyle?
I wanted to feel good again, to wake up energized and ready for the day.

What is your favorite type of workout?
Running (cardio) has become my happy place.

Non-Scale Victory (NSV)!
No more migraines and sleeping better.

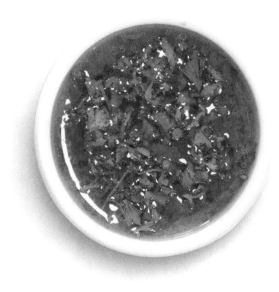

Cilantro Lime Dressing

½ cup extra-virgin olive oil
2 tablespoons fresh lime juice
1 tablespoon apple cider vinegar
1 teaspoon fresh garlic, minced
¼ cup fresh cilantro, packed, chopped
¼ teaspoon sea salt
⅛ teaspoon black pepper

Combine all ingredients in a blender. Blend until smooth. Store in an airtight container in the refrigerator for up to three days.

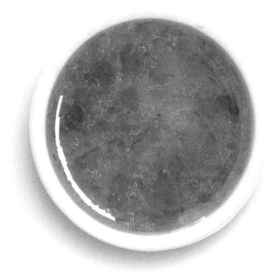

Garlic Lime Dressing

½ cup extra-virgin olive oil
1 tablespoon rice vinegar
1 teaspoon ground garlic
1 teaspoon fresh parsley
1 teaspoon dried dill
2 limes, zest and juice
¼ teaspoon sea salt
⅛ teaspoon black pepper

Combine all ingredients in a mason jar (only the zest and juice from the lime are used), secure the lid, and shake. Store in an airtight container in the refrigerator for up to three days.

E2M Success Stories

Linette A., Danville, VA

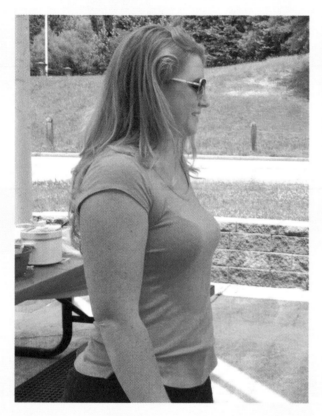 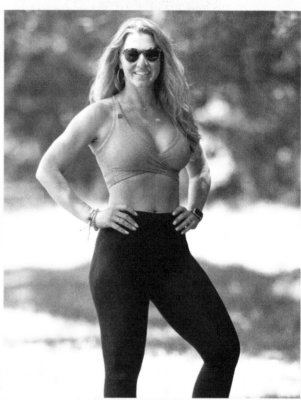

Rounds	Age	Weight Loss
12	36	35

I was eating a line of OREOs® and having a drink every night. I knew I needed to change something and I saw my friend Jessica post her results from the program. We were similar sizes and age and I thought if she could do it, I could do it too. I'm a brand new woman! I've never felt this good physically or mentally. I've gained friendships that will last a lifetime and this E2M community is like no other!

Non-Scale Victory (NSV)!
I have more confidence, I'm comfortable in my skin, and gained lifelong friends.

Spicy Balsamic Vinaigrette

3 tablespoons balsamic vinegar
½ cup extra-virgin olive oil
1 tablespoon Dijon mustard
1 teaspoon ground garlic
⅛ teaspoon chipotle seasoning
¼ teaspoon sea salt
⅛ teaspoon black pepper

Combine all ingredients in a mason jar, secure the lid, and shake. Store in an airtight container in the refrigerator for up to three days.

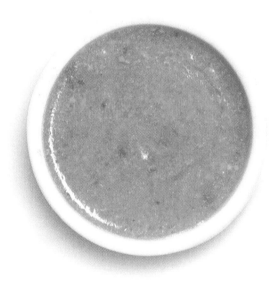

Avocado Lime Dressing

½ cup extra-virgin olive oil
1 avocado, peeled and diced
3 tablespoons lime juice
1 tablespoon apple cider vinegar
¼ cup cilantro, chopped
1 teaspoon Dijon mustard
¼ teaspoon sea salt
⅛ teaspoon black pepper

Combine all ingredients in a blender. Blend until smooth. Store in an airtight container in the refrigerator for up to three days.

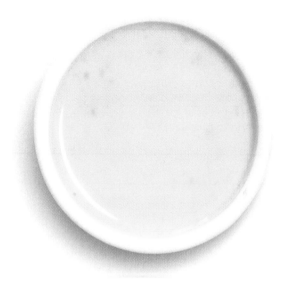

Creamy Tahini Dressing

¼ cup water
¼ cup tahini
3 tablespoons lemon juice
1 fresh garlic clove, minced
½ teaspoon Dijon mustard
¼ teaspoon sea salt
⅛ teaspoon black pepper

Combine all ingredients in a blender.
Blend until smooth. Store in an airtight
container in the refrigerator for up to
three days.

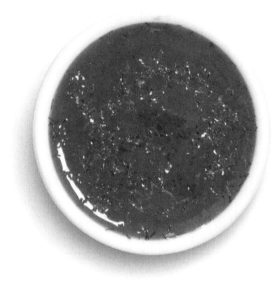

Vegan "Ranch" Dressing

½ cup extra-virgin olive oil
¼ cup rice wine vinegar
1 teaspoon ground garlic
1 tablespoon fresh parsley
1 teaspoon dried dill
¼ teaspoon dried thyme
1 lime, zest and juice
1 tablespoon chopped fresh cilantro
¼ teaspoon sea salt
⅛ teaspoon black pepper

Combine all ingredients in a blender (only the
zest and juice from the lime are used). Blend
until smooth. Store in an airtight container in the
refrigerator for up to three days.

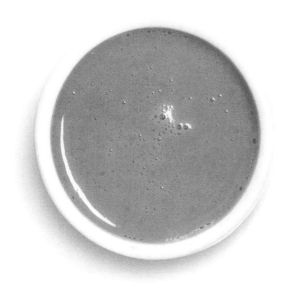

Thai Peanut Dressing

¼ cup peanut butter
3 tablespoons lime juice
1 tablespoon soy sauce
2 teaspoons fresh grated ginger
½ teaspoon chili paste
1 garlic clove, minced
¼ teaspoon sea salt
⅛ teaspoon ground black pepper

Combine all ingredients in a blender.
Blend until smooth. Add water as
needed to thin the sauce to your desired
consistency. Season with sea salt and black
pepper. Store in an airtight container in
the refrigerator for up to three days.

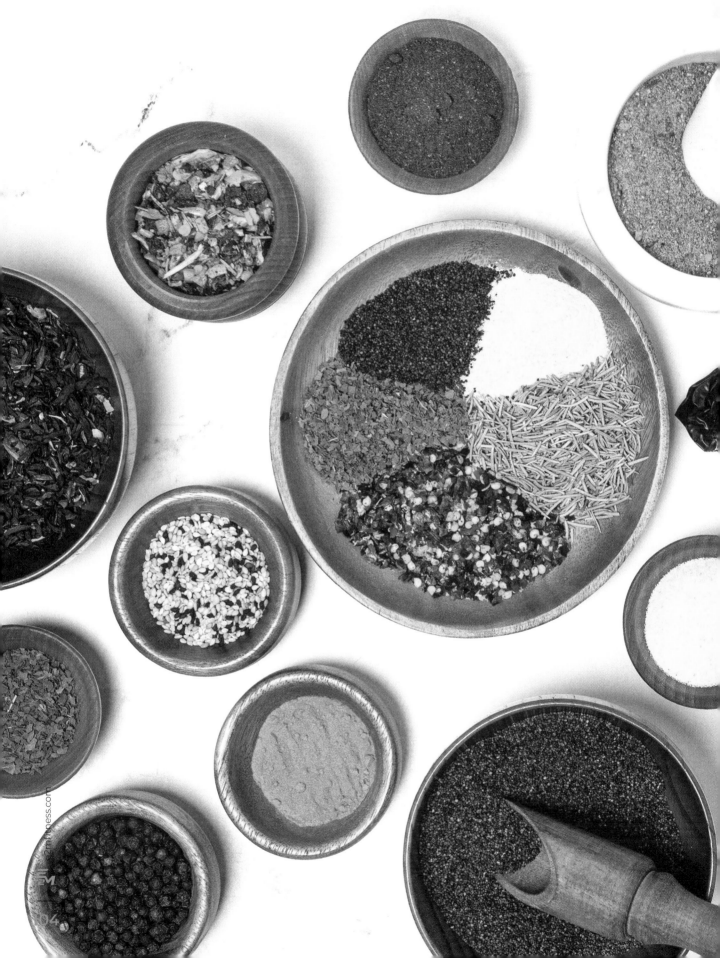

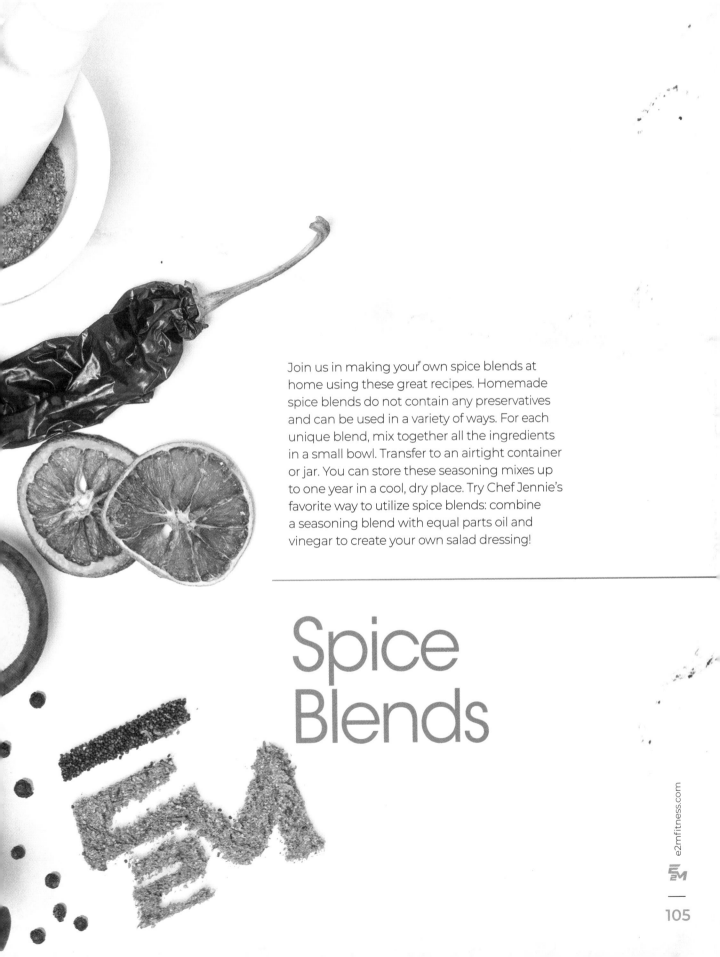

Join us in making your own spice blends at home using these great recipes. Homemade spice blends do not contain any preservatives and can be used in a variety of ways. For each unique blend, mix together all the ingredients in a small bowl. Transfer to an airtight container or jar. You can store these seasoning mixes up to one year in a cool, dry place. Try Chef Jennie's favorite way to utilize spice blends: combine a seasoning blend with equal parts oil and vinegar to create your own salad dressing!

Spice Blends

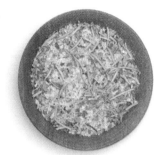

Mediterranean Blend

1 teaspoon ground garlic
½ teaspoon sea salt
½ teaspoon dried rosemary
½ teaspoon dried oregano
½ teaspoon black pepper
½ teaspoon lemon zest

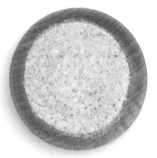

Ginger Garlic Blend

1 tablespoon ground ginger
1½ teaspoons ground garlic
1 teaspoon black pepper
¼ teaspoon sea salt

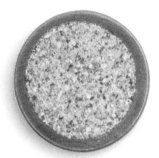

Lemon Pepper Seasoning

1 tablespoon lemon zest
1½ teaspoons ground
    rainbow peppercorn
½ teaspoon onion powder
½ teaspoon ground garlic

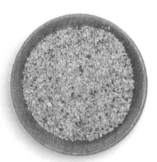

Chili-Lime Seasoning

½ teaspoon dried
    smoked paprika
½ teaspoon ground garlic
½ teaspoon black pepper
½ teaspoon dried oregano
¼ teaspoon ground
    cayenne pepper
1 teaspoon sea salt
1 teaspoon chili powder
1 teaspoon olive oil
Zest from 1 lime

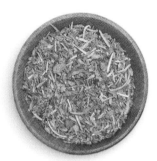

Herbs de Provence Seasoning

1 tablespoon dried thyme
1 tablespoon dried basil
1½ teaspoons dried oregano
1 teaspoon dried rosemary
½ teaspoon dried tarragon

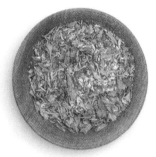

"Ranch" Seasoning

1½ tablespoons ground garlic
1 tablespoon dried thyme
1 tablespoon dried parsley
1 tablespoon dried dill
1 tablespoon dried cilantro
⅛ teaspoon sea salt
⅛ teaspoon black pepper

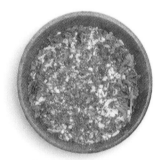

Jerk Seasoning

1 tablespoon ground garlic
2 teaspoons ground
   cayenne pepper
2 teaspoons onion powder
2 teaspoons dried thyme
2 teaspoons dried parsley
2 teaspoons sea salt
1 teaspoon dried paprika
1 teaspoon ground allspice
½ teaspoon black pepper
½ teaspoon crushed red pepper
½ teaspoon ground nutmeg
¼ teaspoon ground cinnamon

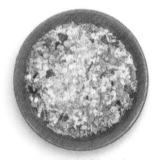

Peri Peri Blend

2 teaspoons dried paprika
2 teaspoons ground
   cayenne pepper
2 teaspoons ground garlic
2 teaspoons dried oregano
1 teaspoon sea salt
1 teaspoon crushed red pepper
½ teaspoon ground cinnamon
½ teaspoon ground cardamom
½ teaspoon ground ginger

E2M Success Stories

Felicia T., Danville, VA

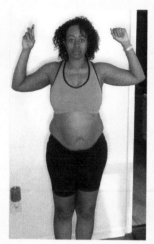 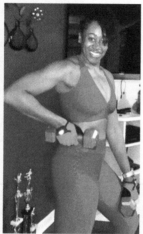

Rounds	Age	Weight Loss
2	40	25

I've always had dreams of being "forty and fit." Well, family (praise break), now I consider myself an athlete. Lol. Yes, I did it! I stuck with it and trusted the process. I am so grateful!

What is your favorite type of workout?
I love the circuit trainings because it gives me the opportunity to challenge myself.

How has E2M fitness changed your life?
I feel ALIVE! I feel powerful and strong! I have prepared my body for whatever life decides to bring.

Joanna J., Dunn, NC

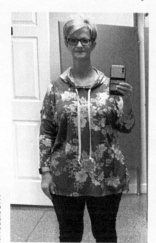 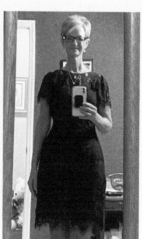

Rounds	Age	Weight Loss
8	59	48

What did you want to change about your lifestyle?
Everything! I just needed simple, straightforward, tell-me-what-to-do instructions with my diet and exercise, and E2M fitness gave me exactly that and much MORE! I had to change my eating and sedentary habits.

What does the E2M community mean to you?
The E2M community is like NO other! It is the most positive, loving, and safe group I've ever been a part of.

Non-Scale Victory (NSV)!
I'm off blood pressure pills.

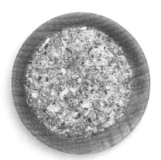

Lemon Basil Seasoning

1 tablespoon lemon zest
1½ teaspoons dried basil
1 teaspoon sea salt
1 teaspoon ground garlic
½ teaspoon dried thyme
½ teaspoon black pepper

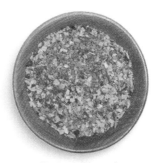

Cajun Blend

2½ teaspoons dried paprika
2 teaspoons ground garlic
1½ teaspoons sea salt
1¼ teaspoons dried oregano
1¼ teaspoons dried thyme
1 teaspoon onion powder
1 teaspoon ground
     cayenne pepper
1 teaspoon black pepper
½ teaspoon crushed red pepper

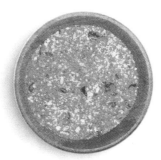

Spicy BBQ Rub

1 teaspoon chili powder
1 teaspoon ground garlic
¼ teaspoon ground cumin
¼ teaspoon ground mustard
¼ teaspoon sea salt
⅛ teaspoon black pepper
⅛ teaspoon ground
     cayenne pepper
⅛ teaspoon crushed red pepper
⅛ teaspoon chipotle seasoning

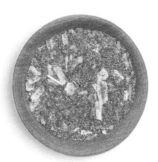

Smoked Chili Seasoning

2 tablespoons chili powder
1 tablespoon dried
     smoked paprika
1 tablespoon ground cumin
1 tablespoon dried oregano
1 tablespoon ground garlic
1 tablespoon onion powder

E2M Success Stories

Joe N., Summerville, SC

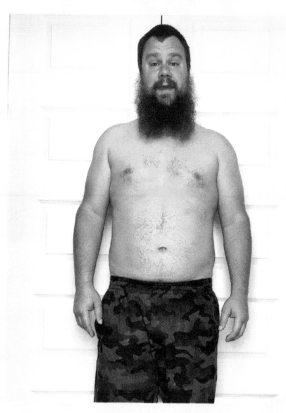 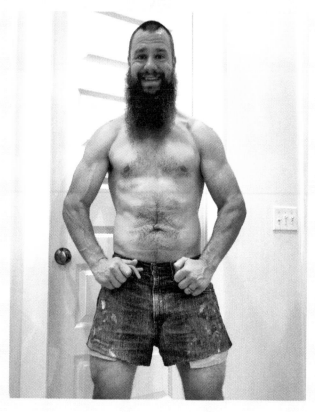

Rounds	Age	Weight Loss
5	**38**	**50**

The E2M program has helped me understand that I have the discipline to achieve and maintain a healthy lifestyle and that becoming physically healthy only requires a small portion of my day with a large return on investment.

What is your favorite type of workout?
My workouts have moved more into a calisthenics-based routine in order to increase strength, fitness, and flexibility with my own body weight.

What does the E2M community mean to you?
The E2M community is where 100K+ of your closest friends are all rooting for you to achieve your health goals.

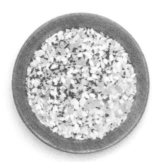

Everything Seasoning

2 tablespoons ground garlic
2 tablespoons onion powder
½ teaspoon poppy seeds
½ teaspoon sesame seeds
½ teaspoon black pepper
¼ teaspoon sea salt

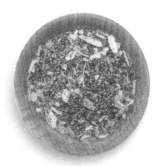

Southwestern Seasoning

2 tablespoons chili powder
1 tablespoon ground cumin
1 tablespoon dried oregano
1 tablespoon ground garlic
1 tablespoon onion powder

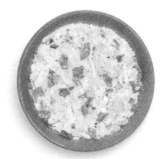

Asian Spice Blend

1½ tablespoons ground garlic
1½ teaspoons sea salt
1½ teaspoons ground ginger
1½ teaspoons crushed red pepper
1½ teaspoons black pepper
1½ teaspoons onion powder

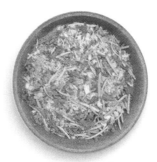

Lemon Herb Spice Blend

1 teaspoon dried paprika
1 teaspoon dried rosemary
½ teaspoon sea salt
½ teaspoon black pepper
¼ teaspoon ground garlic
¼ teaspoon dried parsley
¼ teaspoon ground mustard
¼ teaspoon onion powder
Zest from 1 lemon

Success Stories

Rebecca A., Summerville, SC

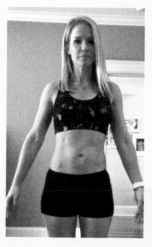
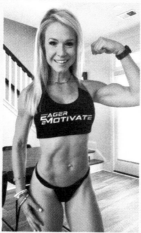

Rounds	Age	Weight Loss
9	38	6

The E2M community was the missing piece of my life. Since joining, I've learned to love who I am, which has allowed me to love and appreciate those around me. I've met the greatest friends here, who I now consider family.

Non-Scale Victory (NSV)!
I'm mentally stronger than I've ever been!

What did you want to change about your lifestyle?
I wanted a more consistent, dependable lifestyle and I wanted a realistic way of living while being healthy and a great influence on my kids.

Chadwick B., Double Oak, TX

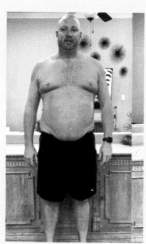
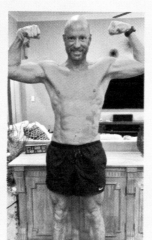

Rounds	Age	Weight Loss
4	48	65

I was hoping to lose fifty pounds, but I received so much more than just weight loss. The internal changes to my confidence and happiness have been dramatic and life changing.

What did you want to change about your lifestyle?
I've done a complete 180 degrees and I am much more efficient with my time because each day has a set of goals that I need to accomplish.

What does the E2M community mean to you?
It means everything to me. It's the special sauce that makes this group so amazing.

Additional
Spice Blends

Buffalo Seasoning

1 teaspoon chili powder
1 teaspoon dried paprika
½ teaspoon onion powder
½ teaspoon ground garlic
½ teaspoon sea salt
¼ teaspoon black pepper
¼ teaspoon ground
    cayenne pepper

Greek Seasoning

2 tablespoons dried oregano
1 tablespoon dried dill
1 tablespoon ground garlic
1 tablespoon onion powder
½ teaspoon sea salt
¼ teaspoon black pepper

Adobo Seasoning

1 tablespoon sea salt
1 tablespoon dried
    Spanish paprika
2 teaspoons black pepper
2 teaspoons ground garlic
1 teaspoon onion powder
1 teaspoon dried oregano
1 teaspoon chili powder
1 teaspoon ground cumin

Veggie Seasoning

3 tablespoons onion powder
1 tablespoon ground garlic
1 tablespoon sea salt
1 teaspoon black pepper
1 teaspoon dried thyme
1 teaspoon dried paprika
½ teaspoon dried parsley

Curry Powder

4 teaspoons ground coriander
2 teaspoons ground turmeric
2 teaspoons ground mustard
2 teaspoons chili powder
1 teaspoon sea salt
1 teaspoon ground
    cayenne pepper
1 teaspoon ground cumin
½ teaspoon ground cardamom

Garlic and Herb
Seasoning

¼ cup kosher salt
1 tablespoon ground garlic
1 tablespoon lemon zest
2 teaspoons dried rosemary
1½ teaspoons dried thyme
1½ teaspoons dried oregano
¼ teaspoon dried paprika
¼ teaspoon crushed
    red pepper

Seafood Spice Blend

1 ½ teaspoons salt
1 tablespoon celery seed
1 ½ teaspoons sweet paprika
1 teaspoon ground dry mustard
1 teaspoon ground ginger
5 bay leaves, ground
½ teaspoon smoked paprika
½ teaspoon freshly ground
    black pepper
¼ teaspoon crushed
    red pepper flakes
⅛ teaspoon ground nutmeg
⅛ teaspoon ground cardamom
⅛ teaspoon ground allspice
⅛ teaspoon ground cinnamon
1 pinch of ground cloves

Thai Spice Blend

2 teaspoons dried paprika
1 teaspoon ground turmeric
1 teaspoon black pepper
1 teaspoon ground coriander
1 teaspoon ground fenugreek
1 teaspoon sea salt
½ teaspoon dry mustard
½ teaspoon ground cumin
½ teaspoon ground ginger
⅛ teaspoon ground
    cayenne pepper

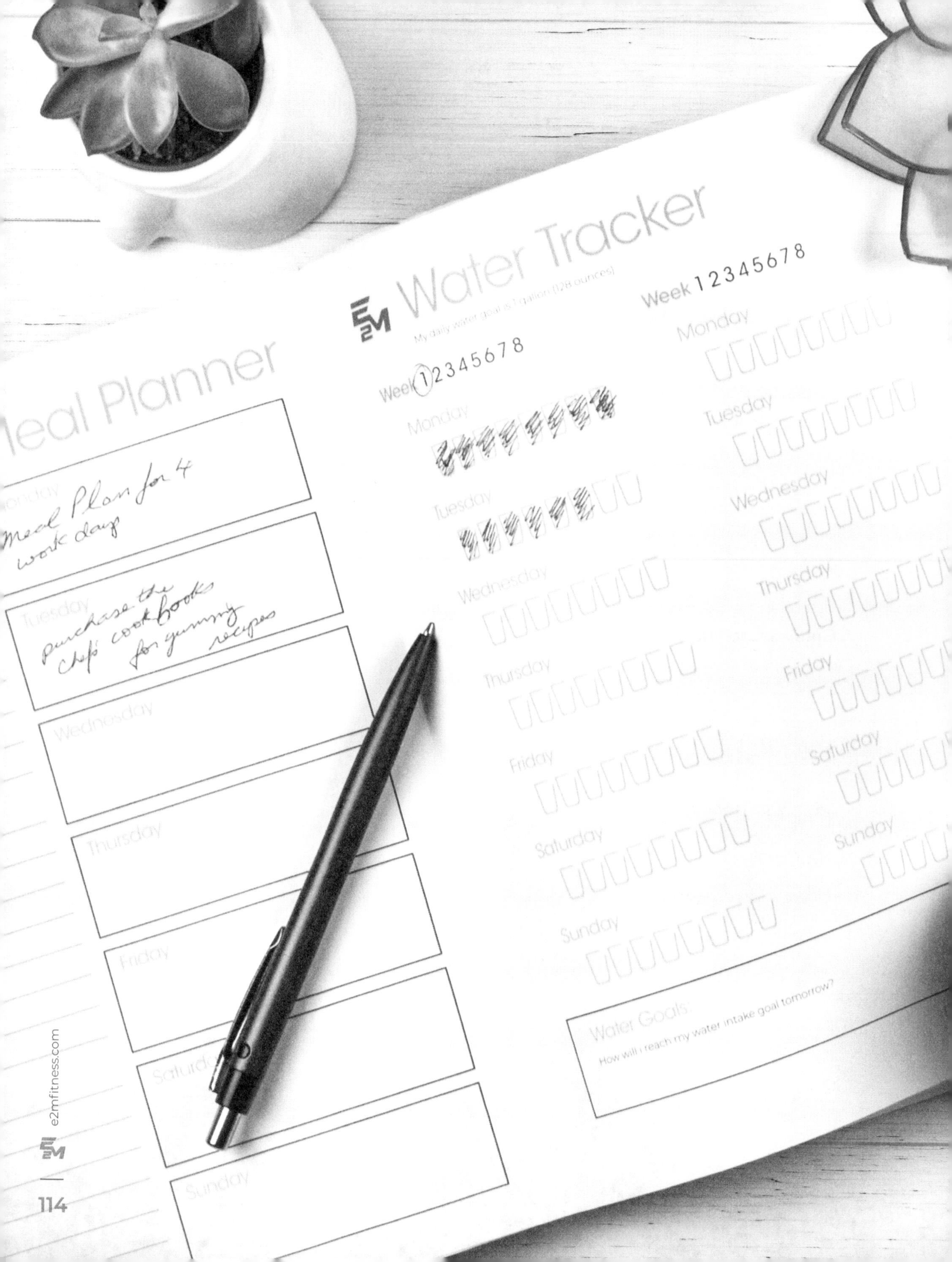

Meal Planner

Monday

Meal Plan for 4
work days

Tuesday

purchase the
chefs cookbooks
for yummy
recipes

Wednesday

Thursday

Friday

Saturday

Sunday

Water Tracker

My daily water goal is 1 gallon (128 ounces)

Week 1 2 3 4 5 6 7 8

Monday

Tuesday

Wednesday

Thursday

Friday

Saturday

Sunday

Week 1 2 3 4 5 6 7 8

Monday

Tuesday

Wednesday

Thursday

Friday

Saturday

Sunday

Water Goals

How will I reach my water intake goal tomorrow?

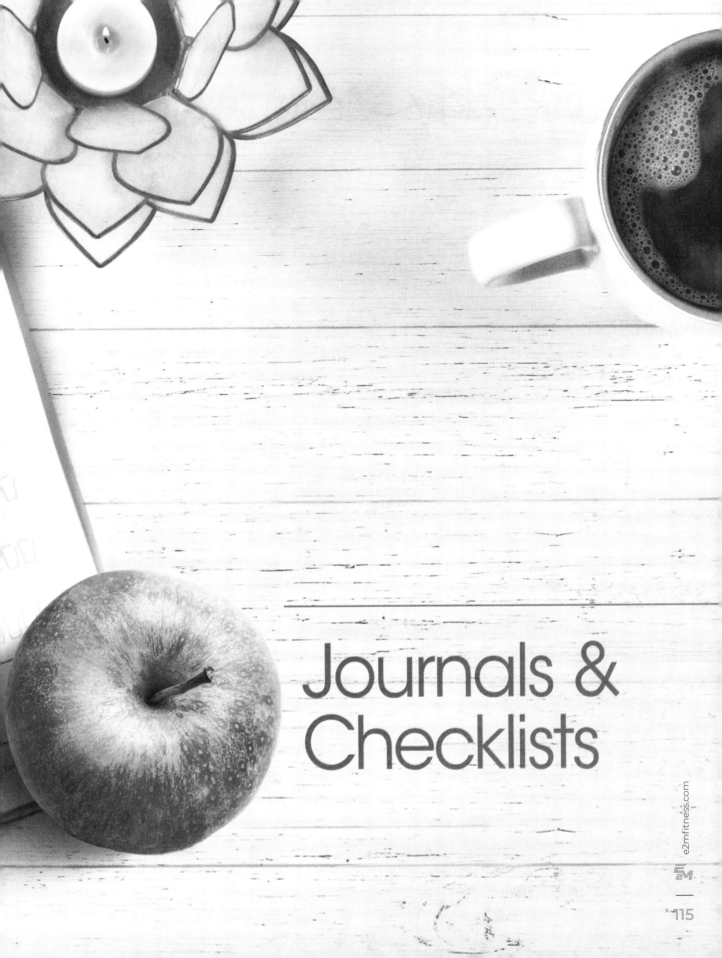

Journals & Checklists

Weekly Meal Planner

Grocery List

Veggies

_____

_____

_____

_____

_____

_____

Protein

_____

_____

_____

_____

_____

_____

Other

_____

_____

_____

_____

Monday

Tuesday

Wednesday

Thursday

Friday

Saturday

Sunday

≡ Water Tracker

My daily water goal is 1 gallon (128 ounces).

Week 1 2 3 4 5 6 7 8

Monday

Tuesday

Wednesday

Thursday

Friday

Saturday

Sunday

Week 1 2 3 4 5 6 7 8

Monday

Tuesday

Wednesday

Thursday

Friday

Saturday

Sunday

Water Goals:

How will I reach my water intake goal tomorrow?

 Each glass represents 16 ounces

Weekly Exercise

Monday	Tuesday

Wednesday	Thursday

Friday	Saturday

Sunday	Non-Scale Victory for the week:
	YAY ME!

Me vs. Me! Trust the Process!

Monthly Habits

Check or color in the square for the new healthy habits you completed.

	Meal Prep	Meal 1	Meal 2	Meal 3	Mental Fitness	Workout 1	Workout 2	Jeff's Live	Water Goal	Celebration Meal	Journal
Day 1											
Day 2											
Day 3											
Day 4											
Day 5											
Day 6											
Day 7											
Day 8											
Day 9											
Day 10											
Day 11											
Day 12											
Day 13											
Day 14											
Day 15											
Day 16											
Day 17											
Day 18											
Day 19											
Day 20											
Day 21											
Day 22											
Day 23											
Day 24											
Day 25											
Day 26											
Day 27											
Day 28											
Day 29											
Day 30											
Day 31											

Weekly Meal Planner

Grocery List

Veggies

_____

_____

_____

_____

_____

_____

Protein

_____

_____

_____

_____

_____

_____

Other

_____

_____

_____

_____

Monday

Tuesday

Wednesday

Thursday

Friday

Saturday

Sunday

Water Tracker

My daily water goal is 1 gallon (128 ounces).

Week 1 2 3 4 5 6 7 8

Monday

Tuesday

Wednesday

Thursday

Friday

Saturday

Sunday

Week 1 2 3 4 5 6 7 8

Monday

Tuesday

Wednesday

Thursday

Friday

Saturday

Sunday

Water Goals:

How will I reach my water intake goal tomorrow?

Each glass represents 16 ounces

Weekly Exercise

Monday	Tuesday

Wednesday	Thursday

Friday	Saturday

Sunday	Non-Scale Victory for the week:
	YAY ME!

Me vs. Me! Trust the Process!

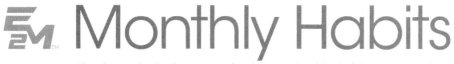

Monthly Habits

Check or color in the square for the new healthy habits you completed.

	Meal Prep	Meal 1	Meal 2	Meal 3	Mental Fitness	Workout 1	Workout 2	Jeff's Live	Water Goal	Celebration Meal	Journal
Day 1											
Day 2											
Day 3											
Day 4											
Day 5											
Day 6											
Day 7											
Day 8											
Day 9											
Day 10											
Day 11											
Day 12											
Day 13											
Day 14											
Day 15											
Day 16											
Day 17											
Day 18											
Day 19											
Day 20											
Day 21											
Day 22											
Day 23											
Day 24											
Day 25											
Day 26											
Day 27											
Day 28											
Day 29											
Day 30											
Day 31											

Weekly Meal Planner

Grocery List

Veggies

_____
_____
_____
_____
_____
_____
_____

Protein

_____
_____
_____
_____
_____
_____
_____

Other

_____
_____
_____
_____

Monday

Tuesday

Wednesday

Thursday

Friday

Saturday

Sunday

Water Tracker

My daily water goal is 1 gallon (128 ounces).

Week 1 2 3 4 5 6 7 8

Monday

Tuesday

Wednesday

Thursday

Friday

Saturday

Sunday

Week 1 2 3 4 5 6 7 8

Monday

Tuesday

Wednesday

Thursday

Friday

Saturday

Sunday

Water Goals:

How will I reach my water intake goal tomorrow?

e2mfitness.com

🏋 Weekly Exercise

Monday	Tuesday

Wednesday	Thursday

Friday	Saturday

Sunday	Non-Scale Victory for the week:
	YAY ME!

Me vs. Me! Trust the Process!

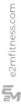

Monthly Habits

Check or color in the square for the new healthy habits you completed.

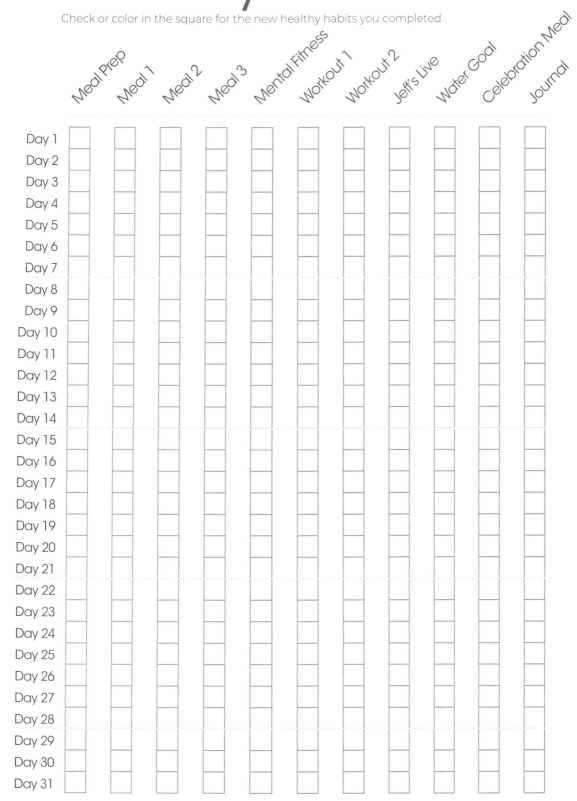

	Meal Prep	Meal 1	Meal 2	Meal 3	Mental Fitness	Workout 1	Workout 2	Jeff's Live	Water Goal	Celebration Meal	Journal
Day 1											
Day 2											
Day 3											
Day 4											
Day 5											
Day 6											
Day 7											
Day 8											
Day 9											
Day 10											
Day 11											
Day 12											
Day 13											
Day 14											
Day 15											
Day 16											
Day 17											
Day 18											
Day 19											
Day 20											
Day 21											
Day 22											
Day 23											
Day 24											
Day 25											
Day 26											
Day 27											
Day 28											
Day 29											
Day 30											
Day 31											